Involving Service Users in Health and Social Care Research

What is the purpose of service user involvement in health and social care research? Can service users go beyond the token gesture and get involved in making a valued and full contribution?

Increasing importance is being placed on service users and professionals being *partners* in services, rather than in traditional roles of provider and recipient. Users and consumers now want to shape their own services and to be involved *in a real sense* in investigations of services delivered, but there is still often a sense of frustration about consultation and involvement being tokenistic and service users' roles being from a position of passivity.

This book takes a more positive and flexible approach and argues that service user involvement in research can range from the extremes of being the subject to being the initiator or investigator of a research study. The activity of the professional researcher can also range from being the person undertaking the research, to being a partner with or mentor to service users. This broad scope of levels of involvement is reflected in the contributions in this book, both in the research experiences reported and in the writing of the chapters themselves. The contributions come from a range of service areas including learning disabilities, cancer care, older people and mental illness, and the chapters look at important research issues such as:

- strategies for working in true partnership
- avoiding 'tokenism'
- involving service users at all stages of the research process
- communication and terminology
- involving service users of different ages and experience
- training needs of professionals and service users
- problems surrounding 'payment' for service users
- other ethical and practical issues.

Involving Service Users in Health and Social Care Research is invaluable reading for researchers in health and social care from academic, professional and service user backgrounds. It will also be of interest to lecturers and students in health, social care and other applied sciences.

Lesley Lowes is a research fellow/practitioner in paediatric diabetes at the Nursing, Health and Social Care Research Centre, School of Nursing and Midwifery Studies, Wales College of Medicine, Cardiff University. **Ian Hulatt** is RCN adviser for mental health nursing, Royal College of Medicine, London.

Involving Service Users in Health and Social Care Research

Edited by
Lesley Lowes and Ian Hulatt

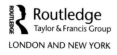
Routledge
Taylor & Francis Group

LONDON AND NEW YORK

First published in 2005 by Routledge
2 Park Square, Milton Park, Abingdon,
Oxfordshire, OX14 4RN
Tel: +44 020 7017 6000
Fax: +44 020 7017 6699

Simultaneously published in the USA and Canada
by Taylor & Francis Inc
270 Madison Ave, New York, NY 10016

Routledge is an imprint of the Taylor & Francis Group

Typeset in Sabon by J&L Composition, Filey, North Yorkshire
Printed and bound in Great Britain by TJ International Ltd, Padstow, Cornwall

British Library Cataloguing in Publication Data
A catalogue record for this book is available from the British Library

Library of Congress Cataloging in Publication Data
Involving service users in health and social care research/[edited by] Lesley Lowes and Ian Hulatt.
    p. ; cm.

    Includes bibliographical references and index.

ISBN 0-415-34646-0 (hardback : alk. paper) — ISBN 0-415-34647-9 (pbk. : alk. paper)
1. Medical care—Research—Great Britain—Citizen participation. 2. Social service—
Research—Great Britain—Citizen participation. 3. Public health—Research—Great
Britain—Citizen participation. 4. Medical care—Research—Methodology. 5. Social service—
Research—Methodology. 6. Public health—Research—Methodology. 7. Patient
participation—Great Britain.

[DNLM: 1. Consumer Participation. 2. Research. W 20.5 I62 2005]

I. Lowes, Lesley, 1950- II. Hulatt, Ian.

RA440.87.G71586 2005

362.1'072'041—dc22

2005004163

Contents

The contributors

Sam Ahmedzai is chair of palliative medicine at the Academic Palliative Medicine Unit, University of Sheffield.

Daphine Aikens is a mother of two children in south-west London.

Meryl Basham is the Torbay 5 A DAY coordinator at Torbay Primary Care Trust, Paignton, Devon.

Peter Beresford is professor of social policy and director of the Centre for Citizen Participation at Brunel University. He is a long-term user of mental health services and chair of Shaping Our Lives, the independent, national user controlled organization.

Krysia Canvin is a research fellow in the Department of Public Health at the University of Liverpool.

Marion Clark is a user researcher at the University of Birmingham and a user of mental health services. In addition to working on other projects since *Cases for Change*, she is currently helping to develop meaningful user involvement in the Heart of England Mental Health Research Network Hub, Birmingham.

Joanne Cook is a senior research fellow for the European Research Area on Ageing, Sociological Studies at the University of Sheffield.

David Cunningham is consultant in oncology at the Royal Marsden Hospital and chair of the Upper Gastro-Intestinal Clinical Studies Group, National Cancer Research Institute (NRCI), London.

Janet Darbyshire is director of the Medical Research Council (MRC) Clinical Trials Unit, London.

Mouse England is a user researcher with learning difficulties who is a member of the Bristol Self-Advocacy Research Group.

Clare Evans is a disabled person with a background in social work and training. She is president of Wiltshire and Swindon Users' Network, and manages the User Empowerment Project nationally for Leonard Cheshire.

Jennie Fleming is principal lecturer (research) and director of the Centre for Social Action, De Montfort University, Leicester.

Jon Glasby is a qualified social worker and a senior lecturer in the Health Services Management Centre, University of Birmingham.

Jennifer Harris is a senior research fellow in the Social Policy Research Unit at the University of York.

Matthew Harris is a research assistant in the Department of Geriatric Medicine, Wales College of Medicine, Cardiff University.

Paula Hodgson is a lecturer in the sociology of health and illness in the Division of Primary Care, School of Population, Community and Behavioural Sciences, University of Liverpool.

Ian Hulatt is RCN adviser for mental health nursing, Royal College of Medicine, London.

Ray Jones has been director of Social Services, and is now director of Adult and Community Services, with Wiltshire County Council. He is visiting professor at the University of Exeter and the University of Bath, and an honorary fellow of the University of Gloucestershire.

David Kirby is a consumer representative at the Upper Gastro-Intestinal Clinical Studies Group, National Cancer Research Institute, London.

Michelle Lake is mother to five children, a meal-time assistant, after-hours activities organizer, parent governor at a local primary school, and an active collaborator on the Watcombe Housing Project, Devon.

Mary Leamy is a senior lecturer in psychology at Teesside University, Middlesbrough.

Helen Lester is a reader in primary care in the Department of Primary Care, University of Birmingham, and has been a general practitioner (GP) in inner-city Birmingham since 1989.

Lesley Lowes is a research fellow/practitioner in paediatric diabetes at the Nursing, Health and Social Care Research Centre, School of Nursing and Midwifery Studies, Wales College of Medicine, Cardiff University.

Hannah Morgan is a lecturer in the Department of Applied Social Science at Lancaster University.

Tina Moules is director of research at the Anglia Institute of Health and Social Care, Anglia Polytechnic University, Chelmsford.

Ruth Northway is a professor of learning disability nursing in the Unit for Development in Intellectual Disabilities, School of Care Sciences, University of Glamorgan, Pontypridd.

Brenda Roche is a qualitative health researcher, currently working on her doctorate in health policy at London School of Hygiene and Tropical Medicine. She is also a policy executive in health and homelessness with Crisis, the national charity for single homeless people.

Phillipa Savile is a former occupational therapist and is a mother of five children in south-west London.

Amy Scammell is the research manager at Wandsworth Primary Care Research Centre, Wandsworth Primary Care Trust, London. She is currently undertaking a doctorate in sociology examining risk assessment and management in forensic psychiatry.

Roger Steel is the development worker at 'INVOLVE' (formerly Consumers in NHS Research), Eastleigh, Hampshire.

Tony Stevens is the consumer liaison lead at the National Cancer Research Network, Cookridge Hospital, Leeds.

Derek Stewart is chair of the Consumer Liaison Group, National Cancer Research Institute, London.

Diane Stockton is mother to five children, has eighteen grandchildren and was a tenant representative in the Watcombe Housing Project, Devon.

The User Focus Monitoring (UFM) group is a group of mental health service users in Wales, who initially came together after being approached by their local health group to collaborate with the local university in undertaking a research project. The UFM group is currently commissioned to undertake further user led research.

Julia Waldman is a senior research fellow in the Division of Social Work Studies at the University of Southampton, and learning and teaching adviser for the Subject Centre for Social Policy and Social Work, part of the Higher Education Academy.

Lorna Warren is a lecturer at the Department of Sociological Studies, University of Sheffield.

Paul Wheeler is a senior lecturer in the Unit for Development in Intellectual Disabilities, School of Care Sciences, University of Glamorgan, Pontypridd.

David Wilde is a research associate at the Academic Surgical Oncology Unit, University of Sheffield.

Val Williams is a research fellow with Norah Fry Research Centre at the University of Bristol.

Dawn Wragg is co-chair of the North Trent Cancer Research Network Consumer Research Panel, Sheffield.

Foreword

Philip Burnard

While research cannot always have a practical focus, it helps, in health and social care, if it does. This is a very timely book and one that I welcome. Although academics and service staff are often involved in research, the consumers often aren't – except as subjects or respondents. This practical book outlines how this might be changed.

The book does not shy away from difficult issues. An example of what might be considered ethically complicated is the involvement of those with mental health problems. The chapter on this is thought-provoking and helpful. Philosophical issues, too, are dealt with in these pages, alongside practical ideas for increasing user involvement. We cannot have a complete picture of what health and social care is about unless we involve consumers.

The book also raises, alongside its text, another issue – that of equality. If we are not careful, as health and social care professionals, we tend to divide the world, unnaturally, into care providers and care consumers. In fact, of course, we are all consumers in one form or another. A book like this, though, raises the question of the degree to which we treat consumers as equals – in our health and social care practice and in our research. While it is clear that consumers come to us with specific needs and requirements and that health and social care professionals have specific skills and knowledge, it should also be clear that *as people* we are all much the same. I hope this book will remind readers of this and encourage them to reflect on their own relationships with consumers.

The editors are to be congratulated on this volume. They have gathered together a range of experienced practitioners and theorists and produced a readable and useful book. I hope that anyone interested in research in health and social care will read it and, in the end, that must include all health and social care professionals, teachers and researchers. It will help to inform research practice and, more than that, it will help all health and social care professionals to reflect on their beliefs and practices. It is a very welcome addition to the literature.

Professor Philip Burnard
School of Nursing and Midwifery Studies
Wales College of Medicine
Cardiff University, Wales

Introduction

Ian Hulatt and Lesley Lowes

As editors, we welcome you to this volume of contributions from the world of service user research, an exciting and developing field of inquiry. We believe that this edited book will prove a valuable resource to health and social care researchers, practitioners and students alike.

What is the purpose of service user involvement in research? The purpose may almost be better expressed as a belief; a core belief that underpins and has consequences for the conduct of research, consequences that are exemplified in the chapters in this book. With increasing importance placed on service users and professionals as partners in the receiving of services, consumers of services now wish to be shaping those services and be involved *in a real sense* in investigations of services delivered. Yet, could it not be argued that the growth of consumerism in health and social care services has already achieved this goal? The advent of consumerism in health and social services was expressed in the United Kingdom by the initiation of benchmarks such as the Charter Mark scheme. The introduction of market principles, such as consumerism, required the introduction of assessing satisfaction with services received. However, this was essentially considered a passive process by service users, who were consulted regarding services but saw no real place for their input in the process of shaping those services. A sense of frustration about being consulted in a tokenistic manner extended further into the arena of research. Service users were involved in research but mainly as subjects, a position of passivity that required their voice to be absent from the shaping of the research agenda or indeed design (for fear of bias). Furthermore, service users, in the absence of some form of feedback, had to wait until publication to see the results of their input. Consumerist approaches to inquiry may well have been a starting point but this has led to a requirement by service users to move further into the area of collaboration, and then to commissioning of research.

Service user involvement can range from the extremes of being the subject (object) to being the initiator and/or investigator of a research study. Similarly, the activity of the professional researcher can range from being the person undertaking the research upon the subject, to being a partner with, or mentor to, service users. This scope of levels of involvement is reflected in the contributions in this book. It is clear, though, that these roles can be fluid; that individuals may shift or fluctuate in their levels of involvement because not only do the needs of research change but so also do the needs of those involved in research. The purpose of service user research can, therefore, be seen within a model of varying levels of involvement.

We believe, therefore, that service user involvement in research should be considered in the context of a *continuum*, as identified in a working paper, *User Involvement in User-focused Research* (Alabaster et al. 2000–2), and discussed by Peter Beresford in Chapter 1. We maintain, however, that one end of the continuum is no better than the other, merely different, with poles of the continuum reflecting the diversity of approaches to service user research. This view is illustrated using a model developed by the editors in an attempt to represent the continuum (Figure I.1).

Integral to this model is an emphasis on the importance of learning and personal development of both professional and service user researchers. For example, therefore, service users who begin their research career at the 'subject' end of the continuum are always potential investigators.

Structure of the book

The chapters in this book are written by service user and professional researchers. Some are written collaboratively and some by individual authors, but each places different emphases on issues identified as important and which have shaped their own approach to service user research. Each chapter will now be briefly introduced.

In Chapter 1, **Peter Beresford** locates the theory and practice of user involvement in research in the broader context of developments relating to user involvement and public participation in public policy and practice. He explores key components that support successful user involvement, different philosophical bases for user involvement and issues raised by (and the relations of) user involvement in the production of knowledge.

In Chapter 2, **Roger Steel** discusses issues surrounding the involvement of vulnerable and often excluded groups of consumers in research and development (R&D), identifying some general principles and ideas that can be applied to a broad

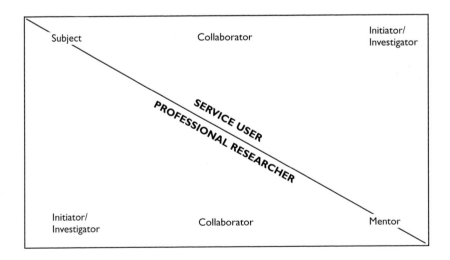

Figure I.1 Continuum model of service user/professional researcher involvement in research.

range of situations. He unpacks and tackles key issues such as 'empowerment', 'marginalization', group 'cultures' and the use of language, payment, consent and advocacy.

In Chapter 3, **Val Williams** and **Mouse England** draw on several inclusive research projects. Including people with learning difficulties in research is often considered paradoxical, difficult or, at worse, a sham. Some concerns and issues discussed in the literature are aired but, primarily, provide a practical insight into how such projects can actually work. The work undertaken to support researchers with learning difficulties is examined in some depth, with ideas gained from an analysis of interaction between supporters and people with learning difficulties.

In Chapter 4, a service user from a **User Focus Monitoring group** discusses the difficulties and barriers of involving people with mental health problems in the research process, from actually setting up a study to the final report. The author (who will remain anonymous) raises issues including the hard fight for service users to be taken seriously and not just used to 'rubber stamp' the process, the 'unfairness' of the process, the 'second class' attitude to service users, the lack of post-research support, and the politics behind the scenes that affected all those involved in the research process.

In Chapter 5, **Paula Hodgson** and **Krysia Canvin** present case studies of a range of models of consumer involvement in research, including consumer led research, research training for consumers, a research steering group, and a workshop to discuss involvement in health research involving users of primary care. Through the comparison of policy guidelines with the reality of everyday practice, they discuss problems related to consumer involvement in health research, including some of the assumptions made about researchers, consumers and consumer involvement.

In Chapter 6, **Jennie Fleming** discusses social action research as a step-by-step methodology that encourages patient/user identification of issues for attention and a continuing active role right through a research project. She introduces the roots and theoretical perspective of social action research and illustrates the application of the approach by describing a research project with a group of foster carers.

In Chapter 7, **Marion Clark, Helen Lester** and **Jon Glasby** describe their experience of being involved in the research process from recruitment of service users to the dissemination of findings. Issues discussed include personal and professional costs, problems created by imposed timeframes, the benefits from service user and 'professional academic' perspectives, and the methods and strategies used to overcome some of the problems that arose.

In Chapter 8, **Brenda Roche, Phillipa Savile, Daphine Aikens** and **Amy Scammell** discuss the involvement of parents as researchers in the context of a study of parents' views about child health surveillance and a health promotion programme offered during the first year of their child's life. Lead parents were involved in all aspects of the research, from participant recruitment to data analysis.

In Chapter 9, **Tony Stevens, David Wilde** and colleagues highlight the growth, nature and influence of consumer involvement in cancer care and research. Opportunities for consumer involvement in research were presented through a cancer network developed through the formation of a Consumer Research Panel (CRP). The authors discuss the organization, structure, financing, operation and evaluation of the CRP, and the recruitment, training and payment of service users.

In Chapter 10, **Meryl Basham, Diane Stockton** and **Michelle Lake** discuss and illustrate the involvement of local people in a community survey of housing and health involving 96 households in social housing in Devon. This resulted in improvements to properties identified in the survey and in a three-year randomized controlled trial. They describe the challenge to continually involve people, and the ethical and methodological issues that this raised during this research experience.

In Chapter 11, **Mary Leamy** provides an honest, reflective account of the experiences of both professional researchers and older people involved in a study exploring housing decisions in old age. Older people were involved in the research process as participants, advisers, commentators and novice researchers. This chapter describes the practical nature and extent of users' involvement, and reflects upon the development, maintenance, renegotiation and continuance of research relationships between users and professionals.

In Chapter 12, **Clare Evans** and **Ray Jones** reflect on ten years of involvement in the promotion of service user involvement in social care. Their involvement in determining the service user perspective through research has resulted in a service user led organization that has been a limited co-operative company since 1993. This company, and its research agenda, has been a key factor in the shaping of policy and practice in the provision of social care.

In Chapter 13, **Tina Moules** discusses the involvement of children and young people in research in the context of a study that set out to explore if and how children and young people could be involved in clinical audit. The chapter highlights the difficulties in recruiting young people to the project, their degree of participation, how they helped to shape the project, collect and analyse data and disseminate findings. Further issues of power, control and resources are discussed, and the chapter closes with a presentation of the views of the young people on their participation.

In Chapter 14, **Julia Waldham** addresses issues that emerged from the practice and evaluation of an innovative new multi-agency, multidisciplinary service for children and young people experiencing severe mental health, emotional and/or behaviour difficulties. The chapter focuses on the realities of how a range of strategies may be used to move the rhetoric into reality and introduces a framework for understanding types of service user involvement.

In Chapter 15, **Hannah Morgan** and **Jennifer Harris** articulate a social model of disability and the development of an 'emancipatory research paradigm', providing a powerful critique of disability research. In the light of this discussion, the authors have sought to devise and develop new strategies for engaging service users at different levels and stages of the project. The authors discuss these strategies, and comment critically on their impact on the management and practice of the research project and the development of new processes within a social services team.

In Chapter 16, **Lorna Warren** and **Joanne Cook** explore service user involvement in research through the experiences of older women volunteer interviewers. They identify a range of ethical issues and consider aspects of service user involvement including recruitment, training, research design, interviewing and dissemination activities. They emphasize the rich potential of involving users in research and policy, and the challenges and adaptation required by those who may be considered professional researchers.

In Chapter 17, **Matthew Harris** discusses a study of the perceptions of older people with Parkinson's disease and their carers about information given. The issues of user organizations as co-applicants and equal partners in research design and data collection, analysis and interpretation are addressed. Using innovative expert round tables comprising patients, carers and professionals (not involved in the research), best practice was identified, and the validity of the findings and improved dissemination were addressed.

In Chapter 18, **Ruth Northway** and **Paul Wheeler** discuss a collaborative research project between a mental health service user group (who initiated the research question) and a university-based academic unit. They explain how the management of the research process promoted a collaborative approach from the stage of designing the study through to dissemination of the results. They identify strategies that were found helpful and lessons that were learnt.

Conclusion

The importance of service user involvement in health and social care research is increasingly being recognized. However, the methodology of service user research is in its infancy and, as the chapters in this book testify, many practical, ethical, methodological and philosophical issues need careful consideration on whatever level of the continuum research is placed. Contributors to this edited volume offer recommendations, based on their own experiences, that address many of the questions and problems that can arise when undertaking service user research. We hope that this book contributes significantly to the advancement of service user involvement in health and social care research. The benefits far outweigh the difficulties for both service user and professional researchers:

> It has not always been comfortable, sometimes it has been particularly challenging, but it has been a win-win for all involved.
>
> (Clare Evans and Ray Jones, Chapter 12)

Reference

Alabaster, E., Allen, D., Fothergill, A., Hanks, C., Hannigan, B., Lowes, L., Lyne, P., Northway, R., Papanikolaou, P., Poole, K., Ryan, J., Webber, I. and Whale, Z. (2000–2) *User Involvement in User-focused Research: A Working Paper*, Cardiff: Nursing, Health and Social Care Research Centre, University of Wales College of Medicine.

Chapter 1

Theory and practice of user involvement in research

Making the connection with public policy and practice

Peter Beresford

The confused context of user involvement

The focus of this chapter is user involvement in research and its relationship with health and social care policy and practice. This means that while the chapter is centrally concerned with research, its discussion also extends to policy and practice. This follows from the view that an understanding of user involvement in research cannot be achieved without some consideration of the role and nature of user involvement in policy and practice. Put simply, we are unlikely to gain a helpful understanding of user involvement in research without consideration of user involvement more generally. Moreover, if the aim is to develop an inclusive approach to 'evidence-based' policy and practice, then we will need to have some understanding of participation in all aspects of the process.

There has been a strong and growing interest in 'user involvement' in health and social care policy and planning since the 1980s. This interest has, however, been slower to develop in health and social care research. While there has been parallel enthusiasm for developing 'participatory' and 'emancipatory' research for much longer, building on ideas and experience generated by community education, feminist and black research, this has tended to develop separately. There has been a tendency for user involvement in research to be treated as a separate entity, without connecting it closely with the lessons learned in the fields of policy and practice.

Why this is, is not clear. It may say something about the broader difficulties that there seem to be in the field of participation, to build on past ideas and experience. The term 'reinventing the wheel' is frequently used in this field. This seems to reflect the problems it has learning from past experience. In one sense, of course, ideas of participation have a history stretching back many centuries to the democratic ideals of ancient Athens. But even understood in much narrower terms, they can be traced to initiatives for public participation going back to the 1960s or so. Yet, so far, there seems to be relatively little to show for this. A recent study highlighted that little if any effort seemed to be made to evaluate the impact of participatory initiatives in the fields of health and social care (Carr 2004). Generally speaking we have little systematic knowledge about what the gains and achievements of participation may actually be.

The frequent failure in research to draw on and synthesize experience of user involvement in policy and practice has other important implications. It is rarely helpful to see research as an isolated area of activity. While there is talk of 'pure' and 'blue sky' research, which is especially committed to the development of knowledge for its own sake, social research is almost invariably policy related and, indeed, often policy reactive. This is particularly true of health and social care research, which are mostly concerned with the theory and practice of provision. If the key role of research is seen as providing the knowledge or evidence base for policy and practice and providing a basis for change, then there needs to be an understanding of the processes involved in achieving this change. We need to know *how* research can successfully impact on policy and practice. While some attention has been paid to this issue, more often it has been overlooked both by researchers and policy makers (Lewis 2001, 2002). However, research needs to be closely connected with policy and practice if it is to play an effective role in policy and practice development and provide a systematic knowledge base for it.

A further issue arises if user involvement is seen as central to the research and policy process. If we accept the current (official) view that change in practice and policy should be based on the involvement of service users, then any efforts to see research as a route to making such change needs to be coupled with some understanding of user involvement in the policy and practice process. Thus, user involvement in research needs to be linked with user involvement in policy and practice development. It is important to be familiar with the issues both raise. The aim here is to help take forward this task.

Involving service users in knowledge-based policy and practice

There are two key sources of evidence or knowledge that have historically tended to be marginalized in health and social care and indeed in public policy more generally. These are the knowledge of:

- *practitioners* – people whose work is mainly face to face with service users
- *service users* – people who are on the receiving end or eligible to receive health and social care service.

Both represent important perspectives and are increasingly recognized as such. Both are at high risk of being overlooked, devalued and ignored. While this discussion focuses on the contribution of service users, this should not be taken to signify any devaluing of the contribution that service workers and their experience has to offer. Practitioner and service user involvement should both be seen as central.

Models of involvement

User involvement is a complex and contentious idea. Certainly, there is little agreement about it. While historically, typologies of participation tended to highlight the *extent* of involvement – most notably with Arnstein's 'ladder of participation' (Arnstein 1969) – the key distinction that now tends to be drawn relates to the ideological underpinnings of different approaches to participation. There are currently at least two key different approaches to or models of participation or user involvement. These may be described as:

- The *managerialist/consumerist approach*, whose focus is the service system and whose concern is to get public, patient and service user input to inform services and provision. This is the predominant model of user involvement in health and social care and has underpinned both state and service system discussions and developments in user involvement.
- The *democratic approach*, whose concern is much more clearly with people's lives and improving their lives; where people as patients, public and service users highlight the need to have more say over the services they use to get the best out of them and to have more say and control over their lives in general. This approach to user involvement has been developed by service users and their organizations but, while it has been influential and has contributed to change, it nonetheless tends to represent a counter-discourse rather than the dominant one (Beresford and Croft 1996).

Each of these approaches is concerned with and promises different things. The managerialist/consumerist approach emphasizes its technicist nature, presented as a neutral means of information gathering. There is no suggestion of any redistribution of power to service users, but this goal lies at the heart of the democratic approach to involvement that is concerned with increasing the effective say and control of service users. Individuals and organizations need be clear about these distinctions when they are making decisions about the kind of user involvement that they want to offer or that they wish to engage with. Problems frequently arise from the failure to do so.

Principles for effective involvement

Like all big ideas, use involvement can readily be subverted. To retain its meaning, user involvement must be recognized as something much more fundamental than the administration of satisfaction surveys, getting people to go to meetings and getting them caught up in the internal workings of the service world. There is no one right way to 'do' user involvement. There is no magic approach that ensures success. There is now, however, an enormous amount of experience to help people get it right, and to get it right as helpfully and cost-effectively as possible. This knowledge and experience has been gained by the hard work of many service users and service user organizations and by supportive workers. There is valuable experience to draw on not only from social and health care but also across public policy and community action more generally (Beresford and Croft 1993).

There is a strong view among service users and their organizations that user involvement must connect with and have meaning in people's lives – both in terms of process and outcomes. In the context of health and social care services, for service users and supportive workers, user involvement tends ultimately to be about improving the treatment, support and service each person gets, so it comes as close as possible to matching what they, with knowledge of what might be possible, might want. Thus user involvement must make a discernible difference in each person's life and experience of service. The acid test of user involvement is that it leads to positive improvements in people's lives and the support and treatment they receive, both individually and generally.

A number of principles for effective and ethical involvement have emerged from existing experience in a wide range of areas. While these do not necessarily offer solutions, there are very few initiatives that have not been informed by or taken notice of the concerns and experience that underpin them, which have been effective.

Support for people to get together

In the fields of health and social care, the importance of supporting the development of service users' own independent groups and organizations was highlighted first and most effectively by the disabled people's movement (Oliver 1996; Campbell and Oliver 1996). While initiatives for involvement are often directed at the individual, support for self-organization – that is for people to be able to get together on their own terms and under their own control – is crucial. The disabled people's movement emphasized the importance of such collective action as a basis for both personal and political empowerment. By supporting sustained opportunities for people in similar situations to get together, it becomes possible to develop an infrastructure for and strategic approach to user involvement.

Coming together in this way, people are able to gain information, gain confidence and skills, develop ideas, bounce them off each other and exert more influence. There must be more support for self-help, support and user groups. These can also provide opportunities for feeding in comments, ideas and proposals for improving policy and provision. Being able to get together, for those who want to, provides essential opportunities to develop collective user involvement to complement the views of patients and service users gained as individuals. It also offers a helpful route for accessing and including non-affiliated service users, since service user organizations have a particular capacity to encourage involvement through the trust and shared experience that they have.

Equal opportunities in user involvement

Initiatives for user involvement need to challenge rather than mirror prevailing exclusions and discriminations. This is still often not the case. User involvement must address difference and ensure that people are involved on equal terms regardless of gender, sexuality, age, disability, distress, class, culture or race. There is talk of 'hard to reach' groups, but this tends to be a euphemism for groups facing particular exclusions and marginalization. There are two particular issues that must be addressed with specific initiatives taken to ensure they are. First, black people, members of minority ethnic groups, refugees and asylum seekers need to be afforded specific support and opportunities to be involved on equal terms. Second, people who communicate differently, whether because they have visual impairments, are deaf or have learning difficulties and do not primarily communicate in writing or verbally, can contribute from their perspectives on equal terms.

Access and support

A key and related lesson about user involvement is that for it to work for *everyone*, there are two essentials that need to be in place. These can be simply headlined as *access* and *support*. Access means that there are structured, ongoing ways of being involved; of engaging with services and agencies, of getting in and connecting with structures of organization, management, control and decision making. Support means that people can expect to have whatever help, support, encouragement, information and skill development they may each need to contribute what they want to, how they want to. If there isn't access, trying to be involved can feel like banging on a closed door. But if there isn't support, only the most confident, experienced and assertive people tend to get involved – and then they can expect to be 'told off' for not being 'representative'! Both components, access and support, are crucial if the aim is to move to more equal and broad-based user involvement.

Ethical issues around user involvement

It is also important not to forget the ethical issues that user involvement can pose, especially where people face real problems and difficulties in their lives. This is an issue that has particularly been raised in relation to the involvement of people who use palliative care services, where service users may be facing life-limiting illnesses and conditions or all the issues posed by bereavement (Small and Rhodes 2000). Service users may have very limited time or other priorities and may be tired and feel unwell. Concerns have been raised that user involvement may become a new orthodoxy and service users subjected to unreasonable pressure to participate. This is clearly unacceptable. There must be choice about involvement. But there are also the ethical issues around *not* involving people.

Here, key issues of support, which were mentioned earlier, and using sensitive and imaginative approaches to involvement, are crucial. We know that generally, most people want to have a say over what happens to them. So far, the signs are that this is no less true of people facing great difficulties in their lives, including, for example, life-threatening illnesses and conditions or bereavement. Choice is what is crucial here. It is also important to give careful consideration to who is intended to be the primary beneficiary of user involvement. If, ultimately, this is intended to be the initiator of the exercise, with service users seen primarily as a source of data or legitimization, then there may well be significant tensions, raising fundamental ethical issues.

Key areas for involvement

In the late 1980s and early 1990s, when user involvement began to be embodied in government legislation and guidance through the Children Act 1989 and National Health Service and Community Care Act 1990, the emphasis was on user involvement in planning services and in individual 'comment and complaints' procedures. Many service users found these two areas of focus difficult to relate to. Planning services was something far removed from the lives of many people. Complaints procedures were problematic, both because they signified that things had already gone wrong, and many people were reluctant to complain about service providers they were dependent on.

In the years that have followed, service users, notably social care service users like disabled people, psychiatric system survivors, people with learning difficulties, older people, looked after young people and people living with HIV/AIDS, have identified other areas to get involved that have seemed more fruitful and effective. These notably include user involvement in education and training, in developing quality standards and outcome measures, occupational and professional practice and developing user controlled services and support. It will be helpful to look at each of these briefly.

User involvement in education and training

A constant message from service users has been that there are few more effective way of changing practice and service cultures than through involving service users in occupational education and training. This has led to the widespread development of 'user led training', 'user trainers' and training for user trainers. Not only does this make it possible for workers to learn from people with direct experience of services and to find out more about what they want from services, but also it makes it possible, sometimes for the first time, for workers to relate to service users in positive and active roles, rather than in the traditionally passive and dependent role of patients or clients. Service user organizations have pressed for this to extend through all aspects of training; from providing direct input in professional and in-service training to being involved in developing course curricula, providing course materials and, indeed, selecting, evaluating and assessing courses and students. All these are now beginning to happen in social care training and education. The British social work qualification, introduced in 2003, requires the involvement of service users in all stages and aspects of the degree (Levin 2004). The challenge is to ensure that such involvement develops coherently and systematically across professions and occupations.

User involvement in developing quality standards and outcome measures

In recent years, there has been considerable political and policy emphasis on improving quality and developing quality and performance indicators and standards in health and social care. Ideas have mainly come from policy makers, practitioners and managers. They have tended to be managerialist and professionally based in inspiration and approach. We know that patients' and service users' concerns and priorities are not always the same as those of service system professionals. Quality and performance can mean very different things to the two groups. Pressure has developed for service users to be involved in both the development of quality standards and outcome measures and in evaluating and interpreting them. The work of Shaping Our Lives, the national independent user controlled organization, on developing user defined outcome measures has signified the beginnings of this process in social care (Shaping Our Lives et al. 2003).

User involvement in occupational and professional practice

There has been a tendency for user involvement to be abstracted and reified as a distinct entity on its own. This separation of user involvement from the mainstream and its association with special meetings, officers and activities may discourage engagement. But all service users by definition connect with practice and practitioners.

Occupational *practice* is a key (but so far often neglected) domain for user involvement. What this means is the understanding and construction of occupational practice as a joint project between service users and workers; that the former can play an active role in structuring and shaping in accordance with their rights and needs. Service users are thus able to feed into and influence such practice through its whole course, as long as they are able and wish to. Concerns that they signal at one stage can continue to influence it throughout its course.

In this way, practice becomes based on seeking the thoughts, views and ideas of service users. It is a systematic process of discussion and negotiation – which is what the best practice has always been. This represents the most direct (and perhaps most effective) expression of user involvement. It also offers an effective route to user involvement in planning and management. Through the systematic collection, collation and analysis of the individual personal views, ideas, knowledge and experience of service users, a key evidence base is provided for the strategic and participatory development of policy and services more generally.

User involvement in developing user controlled services and support

A key but often overlooked area in which health and social care service users have advanced their involvement has been in the development of their own services and support arrangements. The best known of these are the direct payment schemes that disabled people pioneered and that are now embodied in legislation. Growing out of the independent living movement, which is committed to disabled people having the support they need to live their lives on as equal terms as possible as non-disabled people and based on a social model of disability, direct payments put service users in charge of the 'package of support' they need (Hasler et al. 1998; Hasler 2004). Service users have also developed their own collective user controlled services. While these have often been restricted by inadequate and insecure funding, the evidence is that they are particularly valued by service users more generally (Barnes et al. 2000).

User involvement and research

All these areas of activity that have been discussed are concerned with involving and including the knowledge and experience of service users to improve policy, practice and their lives. But we are also concerned here particularly with knowledge or evidence generated specifically through research and evaluation. This brings us to the particular issue of user involvement in research.

There are two points to take initial note of here. The first is whether policy and practice are ever likely to be truly evidence or knowledge based, rather than following from assertion, assumption and conventional wisdom. We may question, despite the rhetoric, how far this is ever likely to be a feasible goal, given the essentially political nature of policy and practice development. Perhaps the realistic aim is to work for provision that is as knowledge based as possible.

The second point is whether service user knowledge can ever be included on anything like an equal basis unless service users and their organizations are themselves fully and equally involved. This is a complex and contentious issue. It is important to remember that service users have long been included in health and social care research as a *data source*, accessed (essentially without their involvement) through surveys and other research methods. Certainly most service user organizations think that service users' involvement is a prerequisite if any notice is to be taken of their experience and ideas – as they understand them.

Common issues

When we explore user involvement in research, it quickly becomes apparent that many if not all the key issues raised by service users about user involvement in policy and practice apply equally to user involvement in research. If we want user involvement to work well in research, then we will need to address those principles identified earlier in this chapter of:

- ensuring support for service users to get together to be involved collectively in research
- developing equal opportunities for user involvement in research
- ensuring access and support to enable a wide range of service users to be involved in research
- addressing ethical issues raised by user involvement in research.

Similarly, the areas for user involvement that service users and their organizations have found particularly helpful to take forward are likely to apply equally in research. These, as we have seen, include developing:

- user involvement in education and training for research
- user involvement in establishing research quality standards and outcome measures
- user involvement in research practice
- user controlled research services and organizations.

In fact, work on all of these has been taken forward by service users and their organizations (e.g. Nicholls et al. 2003; Telford et al. 2003; Evans and Fisher 1999; Evans and Carmichael 2002).

Different approaches to user involvement in research

At the beginning of this chapter, a distinction was drawn between 'user involvement in research' in health and social care (interest in which, it was argued, was a relatively late arrival) and 'participatory' and 'emancipatory' research, in which there was a much longer tradition. It is important now to return to this. Interest in the latter, emancipatory research, can be traced to the late 1960s and early 1970s. It grew from the disabled people's movement and out of strong concerns that the structures, focus and effects of existing disability research were generally damaging and disempowering to disabled people. A different approach to research was pioneered that has come to be called emancipatory disability research. This tradition has also found other related expressions, with the concept of 'user controlled' research and user and survivor research (research by mental health service users/survivors). The accent in all this research has been on a changed and equalized process of research production, with the prime purpose of research seen as the personal and political empowerment of research participants (Oliver 1992; Mercer 2002). This distinction between the origins of user involvement in research and user controlled research is helpful to recall. It seems to mirror the two competing ideological models or approaches to participation more generally, which were discussed earlier – the managerialist/consumerist and the democratic approaches. If the move to user involvement in research reflects the broader interest in participatory initiatives to include the knowledge and viewpoints of service user, emancipatory and user controlled research reflects a commitment to redistribute power in research and for it to serve a democratizing purpose.

While it can be useful to see these two approaches to participation in research as different, it can also be helpful to see them as different ends of a continuum of involvement for service users, from none to complete control. So if we ask the question 'What do we mean by involvement in research and evaluation?', it may mean anything from no involvement to a controlling involvement. For instance, if we are looking at research design and process, involvement can range from:

- service users being responsible for designing the research, including, for example, research questions, data collection and analysis, to
- service users being consulted over the research design and process, to
- service users having no say in the design and process of research.

There are clearly a wide range of degrees of involvement and what must be clear and agreed is, what amount of involvement is on offer and negotiable. This is likely to determine what purpose such involvement can serve and what kind of ideological basis it reflects.

There is also the issue of where involvement is made available. There are many aspects and stages of research where there may be more or less involvement and, again, this needs to be discussed, agreed and decided. So, for example, there may be involvement in:

- originating the research
- determining who benefits from the research
- accountability of the research and to whom is it accountable
- deciding who is the researcher/researchers and who chooses them
- accessing research funding and who gets it
- deciding who controls research funding
- determining research design and process
- dissemination
- follow-up and associated action.

There may be more or less user involvement in any and all of these. As has already been said, what is under discussion here is a *continuum* of involvement. So far there has been relatively little user controlled research, but it is now beginning to happen in earnest – and its advocates have highlighted its validity. Researchers need not think in terms of all or nothing. It is helpful, instead, to work out where realistically they can be and what they can offer in any given research initiative on that continuum and then to be clear about it. At the same time, it is important that user controlled evaluation and research are seen routinely a part of the spectrum of R&D. How else will we know what the right questions are to ask, what the focus of evaluation should be, unless service users and research participants are involved from the start, at the core, at the heart of the project?

Key issues to be addressed

We know now that user involvement in research raises practical questions, like those raised by any kind of user involvement. It tends to mean things take longer and extra costs are involved. But it also raises much bigger philosophical and methodological issues. We are as yet at the beginning of addressing these, but if service user involvement in research is to grow and be taken seriously (rather than treated as an emotional adjunct of 'real' research), we must take this process forward. For example:

- In an age that places an emphasis on evidence-based policy and practice, what status do the views and experience, the knowledge of service users have as 'evidence'? How do we see the relationship of direct experience to knowledge? What issues are raised by the nature of the relationship between experience and knowledge? Does direct experience provide a particularly important basis for knowledge, or is it seen as inevitably biased and qualified?
- How do you move from the experience of individual service users to collective knowledge?
- How do the knowledge claims of service users relate to other knowledge claims? Are they judged to have the same, less or more value?
- What implications do traditional research values of 'neutrality', 'distance' and 'objectivity', and those of 'emancipatory' and 'user controlled' research, have for each other (Harding 1993, 2004; Pawson et al. 2003; Rose 2004; Faulkner and Thomas 2002; Beresford 2002, 2003; Mercer 2002)?

Finally, who is best placed to interpret the experience and knowledge of service users? Is it service users themselves or is it professionals and researchers who can claim distance from them and their experience? But then won't the latter often themselves be subject to and socialized into the values and understandings of the service system and therefore liable to be bias because of this? Can anyone be seen as impartial here?

Conclusion

These are big questions and they require more discussion. We will all have views. They are unlikely to be the same. If the desire is there for user involvement in research, if the aim is to involve the perspectives, the knowledge or, if you prefer, the 'evidence' of service users, it must then also mean involving service users themselves in the process, in one way or another – to some degree. We cannot talk about involving the views and perspectives of service users without directly involving service users themselves. In an age that emphasizes 'participation', partnership, 'empowerment' and the 'active' patient and citizen, it is no longer enough to think about service users as just another data source. The methodological and ethical problems this raises are major. We need to take this debate forward. We need to take user involvement in research forward. Including the knowledge and experience of service users is a crucial basis for practice and policy. But all these goals are likely to be achievable and defensible only if service users and their organizations are centrally involved in the discussions and developments that will need to take place, and if the lessons already learned in the field of participation are more systematically learned.

References

Arnstein, S. (1969) 'A ladder of citizen participation', *Journal of the American Institute of Planners*, 35 (4): 216–24.

Barnes, C., Mercer, G. and Morgan, H. (2000) *Creating Independent Futures: An Evaluation of Services Led by Disabled People*, Leeds: Disability Press.

Beresford, P. (2002) 'User involvement in research and evaluation: liberation or regulation?', *Social Policy and Society*, 1 (2): 93–103.

Beresford, P. (2003) *It's our Lives: A Short Theory of Knowledge, Distance and Experience*, London: Citizen Press in association with Shaping Our Lives.

Beresford, P. and Croft, S. (1993) *Citizen Involvement: A Practical Guide for Change*, London: Macmillan.

Beresford, P. and Croft, S. (1996) 'The politics of participation', in D. Taylor (ed.) *Critical Social Policy: A Reader*, London: Sage.

Campbell, J. and Oliver, M. (1996) *Disability Politics: Understanding our Past, Changing our Future*, London: Macmillan.

Carr, S. (2004) *Has Service User Participation Made a Difference to Social Care Services? Position Paper no. 3*, London: Social Care Institute for Excellence.

Evans, C. and Carmichael, A. (2002) *Users' Best Value: A Guide to Good Practice in User Involvement in Best Value Reviews*, York: Joseph Rowntree Foundation.

Evans, C. and Fisher, M. (1999) 'User controlled research and empowerment', in W. Shera and L.M. Wells (eds) *Empowerment Practice in Social Work*, Toronto: Canadian Scholars Press.

Faulkner, A. and Thomas, P. (2002) 'User-led research and evidence-based medicine', *British Journal of Psychiatry*, 180: 1–3.

Harding, S. (1993) 'Rethinking standpoint epistemology: what is strong objectivity?', in L. Alcoff and E. Potter (eds) *Feminist Epistemologies*, London and New York: Routledge.

Harding, S. (2004) 'How standpoint methodology informs philosophy of social science', in S.N. Hesse-Biber and P. Leavy (eds) *Approaches to Qualitative Research: A Reader on Theory and Practice*, New York and Oxford: Oxford University Press.

Hasler, F. (2004) 'Direct payments', in J. Swain, S. French, C. Barnes and C. Thomas (eds) *Disabling Barriers – Enabling Environments*, 2nd edn, London: Sage.

Hasler, F., Campbell, J. and Zarb, J. (1998) *Direct Routes to Independence*, London: Policy Studies Institute.

Levin, E. (2004) *Involving Service Users and Carers in Social Work Education, Resource Guide no. 2*, London: Social Care Institute for Excellence.

Lewis, J. (2001) 'What works in community care?', *Managing Community Care*, 9 (1): 3–6.

Lewis, J. (2002) 'The contribution of research findings to practice change', *Managing Community Care*, 10 (1): 9–12.

Mercer, G. (2002) 'Emancipatory disability research', in C. Barnes, M. Oliver and L. Barton (eds) *Disability Studies Today*, Cambridge: Polity.

Nicholls, V., Wright, S., Waters, R. and Wells, S. (2003) *Surviving User-Led Research: Reflections on Supporting User-led Research Projects*, London: Strategies for Living, Mental Health Foundation.

Oliver, M. (1992) 'Changing the social relations of research production', *Disability, Handicap and Society*, 7 (2): 101–15.

Oliver, M. (1996) *Understanding Disability: From Theory to Practice*, London: Macmillan.

Pawson, R., Boaz, A., Grayson, L., Long, A. and Barnes, C. (2003) *Types and Qualities of Knowledge in Social Care*, Knowledge Review no. 3, London: Social Care Institute for Excellence.

Rose, D. (2004) 'Telling different stories: user involvement in mental health research', *Research, Policy and Practice*, special issue on User Led Research: 27–35.

Shaping Our Lives National User Network, Black User Group (West London), Ethnic Disabled Group Emerged (Manchester), Footprints and Waltham Forest Black Mental Health Service User Group (North London) and Service Users' Action Forum (Wakefield) (2003) *Shaping Our Lives: From Outset to Outcome – What People Think of the Social Care Services They Use*, York: Joseph Rowntree Foundation.

Small, N. and Rhodes, P. (2000) *Too Ill to Talk? User Involvement and Palliative Care*, London: Routledge.

Telford, R., Boote, J., Cooper, C. and Stobbs, M. (2003) *Involvement in NHS Research*, Sheffield: University of Sheffield.

Chapter 2

Actively involving marginalized and vulnerable people in research

Roger Steel

Introduction

This chapter is based on a 'think piece' originally written for the Empowerment subgroup of INVOLVE (formerly Consumers in NHS Research). The paper then became a consultation document and was published on the INVOLVE website for the purpose of stimulating thought and discussion on the issues surrounding the involvement of vulnerable and frequently excluded people in research and development. Vulnerable and marginalized people have something important to offer through their involvement, not as research participants, but as active partners, collaborators and leaders in research. Without their active input, research that affects them will risk being irrelevant and perhaps even flawed. The *Research Governance Framework* says:

> Research and those pursuing it should respect the diversity of human culture and conditions and take full account or ethnicity, gender, disability, age and sexual orientation in its design, undertaking and reporting. Researchers should take account of the multi-cultural nature of society.
>
> Research [should be] pursued with the active involvement of service users and carers including where appropriate, those from hard to reach groups such as the homeless.
>
> (Department of Health 2001: 15)

'Vulnerability' and 'marginalization' can mean different things to each of us, but the range of people who are often described as 'vulnerable' or 'marginalized' by service providers is large. It may be that some of these people would not describe themselves as vulnerable or marginalized at all. Whether or not you are perceived, or perceive yourself, as vulnerable or marginalized will probably depend on where you are standing at the time, and in relation to who, or what. From whose context are people or services being evaluated? What assumptions arise from the culture of the group, or subgroup, we belong to? For example, travellers may see the National Health Service (NHS) as hard to reach and marginal to their culture. Any social or organizational group is a single context and can be seen to have its own culture.

The following list includes *some* of the groups who may be occasionally or frequently excluded from involvement in research *because* they are perceived to be vulnerable or difficult to reach by the research community. The list is not an attempt to be comprehensive, but serves to give an example of the range of people who are often described as, or who might describe themselves as, vulnerable or marginalized:

- people experiencing mental health problems/personality disorder
- people with brain injuries
- children in general
- children in care
- young carers
- carers in general
- people with a learning difficulty
- ethnic minorities
- asylum seekers and refugees
- travellers
- homeless people
- frail older persons
- older persons in general
- people experiencing forms of dementia
- people for whom speech and/or hearing is not their principal means of communication
- visually impaired people
- people suffering from a life-limiting illness
- people whose voices cannot be heard
- disabled people
- drug addicts
- single parents
- people who cannot read or write in English
- people who cannot speak or understand spoken English well
- people in poverty
- people who need, but are not receiving, health or social care services
- people whose lives are affected by the complex repercussions of disability, long-term illness, or social care needs, who encounter different services that do not 'join up'
- people in receipt of forensic mental health services
- prisoners.

For the purpose of this chapter, it would be impractical to go into every detail of every practical, social, ethical and legal consideration needed to include all groups of vulnerable or marginalized people in research. Every situation is different, and individuals are different in the scope of their needs and abilities no matter which category or group best describes them. Further, there are also people whose experience of vulnerability can be temporary and circumstantial. Indeed, some of the discussion that follows is probably pertinent to *any* person who *feels* vulnerable or marginalized when joining a research group. A generic approach that is concerned with the awareness needed when engaging with vulnerable and marginalized groups and individuals may be the most helpful. Let us start by unpacking some principles and ideas associated with the idea of inclusion, marginalization and vulnerability.

General principles: inclusiveness and empowerment

Actively involving the public in research is about inclusiveness and, whichever way we look at it, we are asking a group or individual to 'join in' a recognized process involving a 'culture' and context we broadly call the research community. This may involve service users being actively involved on a variety of panels, committees, planning or steering groups. All of these are groups of some form or another, each capable of having its own culture.

Inclusiveness

What do we mean by inclusiveness? We cannot assume that we have included someone in a group or organization until such a time as *they* feel able to contribute as fully and equally as they would wish, within the overall group purpose or terms of reference. To be included is to have an equal opportunity to have one's individual perspectives and needs accommodated, absorbed and integrated by the group or organization.

A research group that decides to recruit a service user on a panel because it is perceived to be 'good practice', but does not otherwise change its practice, is not going far enough. Tacking on someone from the 'outside' because it seems expedient to do so, is not inclusion. This is tokenism. To accommodate a new element, the whole dynamics of any process/structure must necessarily shift as a whole to some degree. It is this ability to shift, which determines the inclusiveness, or the lack of it, in an organization or group. In other words, an organization or group must be prepared to adjust its processes, attitudes and dynamics if it is to properly include a new participant. This is often done unconsciously to a degree anyway, although not necessarily adequately. It is therefore imperative that this adjustment is as conscious a process as possible when it comes to involving potentially vulnerable or marginalized people. The following extract describes 'The Travellers Project', a project about sexual health services used by New Age travellers:

> This project was among the first to involve users following the launch of the national R&D strategy, so there were few examples to which those involved could refer for guidance. However, the difficulties which emerged during the course of the project are not unique to research involving service users. Many might equally arise in any project involving a range of stakeholders with differing expectations, values and experiences. Such is the nature of collaborative and participatory research. While risking over simplification, many of this project's difficulties stemmed from poor communication and a failure to openly and honestly address the fundamental issues of power, accountability and mutual responsibility.
>
> (Woodward and Matthews 2000: 28)

An illustration of inclusiveness in relation to vulnerable individuals is the 'ladder of participation' (Arnstein 1969), depicted in Figure 2.1 (Hart 1992).

Here it serves to demonstrate ways of being involved that any vulnerable adult might experience, and the process of climbing the ladder illustrates the type of adjustment that might be needed by all concerned. The example takes us from a group of

Top of ladder

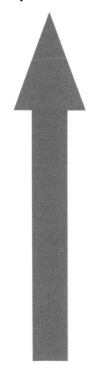

→ **Child initiated and directed** – The children have the idea and decide how they want to carry the project out. Adults are available but do not take charge.

→ **Child initiated: shared decisions with adults** – Children have the ideas, set up the project and invite adults to join with them in making decisions.

→ **Consultation and information** – Adults may have developed the initial idea, but the children are involved in every step of the planning and implementation. They are listened to and are actively involved in taking any decisions.

→ **Assigned but informed** – The children are asked to take part in a project which the adults have designed. The children understand the project and know who decided they should be involved and why. Their views are taken seriously.

→ **Tokenism** – Children are asked to say what they think about an issue. However, they have little choice about the way they express their views or about how frank they can be about any concerns. They may not know what will be done with any views they express.

→ **Decoration** – The children are part of an event. They may sing, dance, listen, but again they do not really understand the issues of the purpose of the event.

→ **Manipulation** – Children do or say what adults suggest they do. They have no real understanding of the issues, although they may be asked for their views. They do not know what influence their views will have on any decisions that are made.

Bottom of ladder

Figure 2.1 Ladder of participation.
Source: Hart 1992.

'vulnerable' individuals being manipulated at the bottom of the ladder to levels of involvement where they have degrees of empowerment and 'ownership' of a project or process. Ownership and empowerment need not always involve total control of a process. It can mean an interest, will and ability to participate and share control and responsibility with others for a mutual purpose. This is interdependence.

Assumed paternity within a group culture can become a major barrier to any involvement, and can be actively excluding, indifferent, or even dangerous to other stakeholders. The Royal Liverpool Children's Inquiry Report (Redfern 2001) is a record of this happening in a health research culture. Whatever the level of vulnerability of an individual, and whatever responsibilities others may have in relation to them, that individual has a right to have information, to make informed choices, to express their views, and, at the very least, have them actively taken into account.

An organization or group needs to actively facilitate an individual with the information and means needed for them to be a full and effective participant. The individual can be enabled to take part and to meaningfully contribute by being armed with an awareness of the purpose, needs and perspectives of the group or organization. Without this, there can be no effective dialogue. The idea of an information pack is an example of how this might be achieved. Mentoring by an experienced group member can be another powerful way of facilitating involvement. Having the appropriate information to know how, why and what to do is one of the ways in which empowerment of the individual comes about.

Empowerment

'Empowerment' is a word open to a range of interpretations, and used to support a range of agendas in public, voluntary and private organizations. The idea that we can 'empower' others is a contradiction in terms. An environment can be created in which individuals can empower themselves, but empowerment cannot be 'done' *to* someone. Fundamental to empowerment is the opportunity to exercise individual choice and take effective action. The barriers that might prevent this can be removed in so far as those who represent the dominant culture of a group are aware that there is a problem, and to the extent that they themselves are willing and able to make changes. However, they can achieve this only in so far as the structure and culture they themselves are obliged to work within allows. For this reason, empowerment is everyone's issue, and needs to be addressed at all levels. To take this on board is to see empowerment as a process in which we must all be actively involved in order to achieve the best possible outcomes for others and ourselves in any given situation.

Marginalization

Those who are marginalized are outside the dominant culture of a group. This could be a professional or social group, or a whole society. An individual may be marginalized out of choice, but more often it is because the dominant culture is unable to accommodate a particular group or individual. Every group has its tolerances and intolerances whether overt or covert, conscious or unconscious. In society, the law generally defines conscious intolerance more or less successfully. Covert and unconscious intolerance can take the form of prejudice and unequal opportunity even if this is against the law. The same covert or overt dynamics apply whether the behaviour is that of an individual or a whole group. The latter might be a research steering group, a representative group of professionals, or service users and any of the organizations within which they operate. Exclusion can be active or passive. Where it is active, it is likely to be conscious or unconscious intolerance. When passive, it is more likely to be about conscious or unconscious ignorance. Whether overt or covert, institutional or individual, the attitudes of others generally have a strong effect on a vulnerable individual and can therefore be fundamentally empowering or disempowering. Such attitudes can be subtle or obvious.

Everyone has needs. We have general needs that we tend to have in common with others and are more or less fulfilled by the way we live from day to day. We also have 'special' needs that make us different, but which we all have from time to time and some people have all the time. A common occurrence in the health care field is when an individual's general needs, which they have in common with any other human being, are overlooked or ignored because attention goes solely on their special (health) needs. For example, we may experience conditions as less than 'human' when we are waiting for hours in an overstretched Accident and Emergency Department for treatment for an injury (special need). But this is where attention to general needs is usually only temporarily suspended. Where special needs are attended to exclusively over a sustained period, it can eventually lead to chronic institutionalisation, marginalization, loss of 'humanity' and self-esteem. In extremes, an individual can become identified only in terms of special needs to the exclusion of all else, and lose their commonality and, therefore, connection with others. This can be the effect of institutional attitudes. Everyone is subject to institutional attitudes to some degree, but for some the effects are more fundamental and 'disabling' than for others:

> For many years doctors, social workers and other people have told disabled people that they are disabled because of 'what is wrong with them' – their legs don't work, they can't see or hear or they have difficulty learning things, just to give a few examples. This is known as the medical model of disability. It says that it is the person's 'individual problem', that they are a disabled person. What we say is that yes, we do have bits of us that don't work very well, this we call impairment: for example, a person who cannot hear very well has a hearing impairment. What we say is that it is not this impairment which makes us disabled. Society does not let us join in properly – information is not in accessible formats, there are steps into buildings, people's attitudes towards us are negative. So society puts barriers before us which stop us from taking part in society properly – it disables us. This is known as the social model of disability.
>
> (Young Disabled People's Group 1996)

In relation to a research project, Users' Voices, the following example demonstrates how practice was changed to include a vulnerable group, and counter the effects of medical attitudes:

> The key to any UFM (user focussed monitoring) work is a local group of service users. . . . The first step for the project co-ordinator is to recruit group members. This involves going to day centres, work projects, and so on. . . . Some people in these settings are immediately interested in getting involved. At the same time, we are often met with many that lack self- confidence. A majority of users in these initial talks think that the project is too difficult for them. Overcoming this lack of self-confidence is a task that continues throughout the life of the project. We have come to the conclusion that mental health services are very good at telling people what they cannot do. On a more positive note, it is almost always the case that those who begin the project go on to complete their work.
>
> (Rose 2001: 15)

A question any of us can ask ourselves is, what makes *us* flourish and participate to the full? What attitudes and processes are helpful or unhelpful to us? Which are encouraging and discouraging, and can we do anything about it? When do we feel included or excluded? What might affect us in health and strength, and to which we probably adapt without thought, can be a major barrier for someone who is vulnerable. Being aware of how different attitudes, environments and processes affect us can help us anticipate potential effects on others, provided we understand that these effects are not always the same for everyone. We also need to be prepared to inquire and learn.

What does this mean in practice?

I have discussed some principles which may helpfully steer us in the right general direction. Principles describe the 'magnetic north' of where we should be heading. On their own, however, they do not describe each step of the way. What practical considerations are needed to help apply these principles? What follows are some suggestions for addressing some of the core practical considerations when involving vulnerable and marginalized people. (For more specific information on involving people with different needs in shaping services, an excellent but lengthy guide is *Asking the Experts: A Guide to Involving People in Shaping Health and Social Care Services* (Baulcombe et al. 1998) available from the Community Care Needs Assessment Project website: **http://www.ccnap.org.uk**.)

Time and resources

Where vulnerable individuals are concerned, it is important to ascertain their needs well in advance. For example, it may be important to arrange for a translator, support worker, signer, advocate, guardian or nurse to be present with them if they so choose. Matters like religious belief may affect arrangements, such as the date of a meeting. All these take time to arrange. Additional time might be needed during a project too. Where relevant, for example, allow time for things to be explained, medication and comfort breaks. It is important to continually check that individuals are able to participate as much as they would wish, and to be prepared to resolve problems that are both anticipated and unanticipated. For example, some disabled people have difficulty in getting to meetings first thing in the morning, and may need to leave because they are tired by mid afternoon, so a meeting in the middle of the day in this case would be appropriate.

Expenses need to be paid, and it should be borne in mind that for a 'vulnerable' person expenses may be higher than usual. Offering payment for time should also be taken into consideration, particularly with groups on low incomes. This can help reduce some of the barriers of financial inequality within the research group. Many vulnerable and marginalized groups will be in receipt of state benefits, and great care should be taken when making payments in these circumstances. This and other important issues of payments is covered in more detail in *A Guide to Paying Members of the Public who are Actively Involved in Research* (Steel 2003), and *A Fair Day's Pay* (Scott 2003).

More time and resources are needed when actively involving vulnerable or marginalized groups in research. We should, however, continually remind ourselves of the end value of this involvement to research and to those we are involving. It will be important to include all of these resource considerations in any proposed research prior to applying for funding. Not only will the budget need to be appropriate, but also the timescales for the research need to be realistic. The research will take longer, and you may also need to plan for a realistic lead in period before the actual research starts, to allow for developing relationships and building trust.

Choice about getting involved

In any instance, when intending to actively involve vulnerable individuals in research projects they must have the opportunity to give their *informed* consent. In other words, as far as possible, the people you want to involve must be made aware of the issues surrounding the choices they are making, including the expectations, consequences, potential pitfalls, and benefits, as well as the alternative options open to them. They will also need to know why the research is relevant to them, and the likelihood that it will make a positive difference to their lives. People will need to be informed in a way that they are able to relate to, and have the opportunity to ask questions.

If an individual you would like to involve is by law a dependant – a child, or someone under legal guardianship or Court of Protection – then the consent of the appointed legal guardian must be sought in addition to that of the child or person under guardianship or protection. If the individual is subject to a legal order, such as a Mental Health Act section or probation order, then the general rule is that consent must also be sought from the officer responsible for enforcing the order. When approaching children or vulnerable individuals, they may need an opportunity to think about whether they want to become involved, and time must be allowed for this. Further, the way children are approached will of course depend on age, and information needs to be conveyed in a way that is acceptable to them and can be readily thought through. Often the approach will be made through a parent or carer in the first instance. The children or vulnerable adults need to be able to make a clear choice for themselves. It is important to ascertain that the choice is theirs and not one made to please a guardian. The children or vulnerable persons will need to be sure they can independently and safely say 'no' or 'yes' in any given situation.

Inclusion in research meetings

Research groups need to be prepared to make adjustments to accommodate the level of knowledge and level of learning ability of the individuals involved. In meetings, those in the role of chair have a responsibility to ensure everyone has an equal opportunity to participate. The group, and particularly the chair of the group, needs to be proactive in ensuring that members are aware they can ask for clarification of anything they do not understand and have the opportunity to do so. In some cases an advocate, support worker or mentor can be helpful to an individual. If they wish it, someone of their choice should work with them. 'Ground rules' for meetings can be agreed by all involved when starting a new research group. These can then be written down so that expectations about how the group will operate are clear. This might best be negotiated at the first meeting. For example, a ground rule could be to 'respectfully listen to another's point of view even if you disagree with it' and/or 'to observe the confidentiality of any disclosure by a group member'.

Sometimes a 'job description' can be helpful in clarifying expectations on all sides. Job descriptions are best created for all collaborators in a research group rather than just for the service users involved. For established professionals, of course, the job description would relate specifically to their role in the group, not their wider remit. For service users, it might, among other things, refer to their responsibilities in giving an independent perspective. For all members, it might refer to the expectation of transparency when stating views, for example, by stating whether they are personal or organizational.

A mentoring system might be helpful for new members in a research group in understanding the issues being discussed or the processes being followed. A mentor could be an experienced member of the group who takes responsibility for making sure the new members are able to participate as fully as they would wish. For long-term groups, a rolling membership is likely to be healthy, provided there is some over-lap. Overlap with an experienced service user member of the group and an incoming service user member could be very supportive where vulnerable and often marginal-ized individuals are involved. It also provides opportunities for more vulnerable indi-viduals to get involved over time, and helps promote an equal opportunities ethos. Be aware that sometimes problems can arise for an individual when leaving a group. For example, it may be quite traumatic breaking away from something you have been personally involved in over a period of time.

Advocacy

The importance of independent advocacy cannot be understated. Whereas an advo-cate cannot override the decision of a legal guardian, they can ensure that the indi-vidual concerned has a 'voice'. The advocate's role is to represent the interests and views of the individual as if they were their own. To do this, a period of time is needed for the individual and advocate to work together to get to know each other, to dis-cuss the issues and build trust. The advocacy relationship should be empowering, in that the advocate does not do all the talking but ensures that where they feel able, individuals can speak up for themselves. Advocacy services are generally local. Some specialize in people with specific support needs and others are generic. Some areas may not have an advocacy service at all. A research group may however be able to identify potential advocates themselves.

Reaching marginalized groups

UK national and local popular media can be powerful in ignoring certain groups of people or in steering public opinion against them. It follows that popular media may not be the best route in reaching those groups unless through a specialized magazine or programme devoted to them. Probably the best way of reaching these groups is through local networks. Including marginalized people in research requires a tena-cious, proactive, yet sensitive approach. There should be a readiness to explain to the groups concerned the value of the research, and the value of their involvement in it, honestly and openly. People are likely to want to know what the benefits are to them, both as individuals, and as groups. Not only is this important in reaching and engag-ing with these groups, but also it is important when enabling them to participate once recruited. It is vitally important to be proactive in anticipating specific needs and to remove as many barriers to meaningful participation as possible. This may take extensive dialogue with the groups concerned.

There is a range of possible routes for reaching marginalized groups but, by defi-nition, some groups are more difficult to reach than others. However, how 'difficult' this seems depends on how hard you are prepared to try. A useful route is to utilize local networks in the community in the statutory sector (i.e. local councils), but especially in the voluntary sector. Community Voluntary Services (CVS), which are 'umbrella' support organizations for local voluntary groups, usually have good information on a whole variety of voluntary group activities across their area. Local libraries and community centres are often a good source of local information, and may have newsletters or leaflets from relevant groups. There may also be a national organization that may be able to help or to signpost your enquiry to the appropriate people. There are databases of both national and local organizations that are an effective start, but sometimes footwork such as attending relevant forums, conferences and gatherings can be necessary to reach a particular group. Word of mouth local networking can sometimes be the only way, and enlisting the help of local community leaders can be fruitful. Remember, some marginalized groups may not traditionally use literature or have the reading or language skills to respond to leaflets or advertisements.

Having located the groups concerned, it is important to ensure that their infrastructure is appropriately supported and not drained by your work. Networks need maintaining and that usually means ongoing resources are needed, whether this is transport, a newsletter, time, postage and telephone costs, appropriate venues to meet, and so on.

Use of language

Clearly, problems arise when language is developed and used to tackle complex specialized issues, such as in research. Whereas it is principally used with the positive intention to produce effective services, specialized language is by definition marginalizing for the non-specialist. It is important, when using specialized terms in the presence of non-specialists, to be conscious of whether meaning is being conveyed in the most effective way for the purpose of the group. Again from the *Research Governance Framework* 2.4.1:

> There should be free access to information both on the research being conducted and on the findings of the research, once these have been subjected to appropriate scientific review. This information must be presented in a format understandable to the public.
>
> (Department of Health 2001: 13)

Despite some important improvements since the late 1990's, health, social care, and academic institutions still sometimes produce information in language that can be difficult even for many educated white middle class people to grasp, let alone those who are vulnerable or marginalized. In research groups, if the issue of specialized language is not addressed, there is a great danger that involving non-specialists will be tokenistic. Service users in research must at least have the opportunity to broadly understand the issues being discussed, as well as the associated papers. Information must therefore be communicated in a way that people can understand. This might be achieved through simple practical measures such as asking a researcher to produce a lay summary of a research proposal that summarizes the paper in a language accessible to all. It may be necessary to put this on tape, have it read and explained or have accompanying pictures that help explain things. There is likely to be a need for 'ground rules' about how people will communicate with each other in meetings.

Conclusion

Improvements in the way a group operates in order to incorporate the views and needs of a vulnerable or marginalized individual are likely to help every group member in the long term. Although it may mean that additional thought, preparation, time and money is needed, it is also likely to mean that the project becomes more effective in terms of its overall aims. Making the dynamics of partnership easier in order to include a vulnerable or marginalized individual is likely to mean that everyone finds it easier in the longer term, even if having to operate in rather different ways. Vulnerable or marginalized individuals are likely to be embarking on an activity that is new to them, and in doing so, making many adjustments. They will be on a learning curve that may at times be uncomfortable. It is not much to ask other members of the project to make adjustments themselves, and be willing to learn new ways of approaching partnerships for the purpose of an effective piece of research.

There is no single 'prescription' for how involving vulnerable and marginalized people should be done. We need to be aware of the issues bearing on each situation and be proactive in addressing them. We need to be able to adjust and learn. We need to be willing to learn from what has been done before, to throw out what does not work and experiment with what might. Above all, we need to be able to value all as equals and experts in their own experience.

People become vulnerable and marginalized for a reason. Sometimes the causes are subtler than we at first realize. There are often complex combinations of inter-dependent factors bearing on each individual or situation. Tackling the causes once they are identified may mean re-examining the fundamental beliefs behind our institutions. Involving vulnerable and often marginalized groups is therefore likely to be a challenge for all, both inside and outside research. Ultimately, this should empower all involved, even if the process of getting there is difficult and perhaps uncomfortable.

Acknowledgements

With special thanks to Kate Sainsbury, Jabeer Butt, Mary Nettle, Deborah Tallis, and Russell Hamilton of the Empowerment subgroup, INVOLVE (formerly Consumers in NHS Research).

References

Arnstein, S. (1969) 'A ladder of citizen participation', *Journal of the American Institute of Planners*, 35 (4): 216–24.
Baulcombe, S., Hostick, T., New, T. and Pugh, H. (1998) *Asking the Experts: A Guide to Involving People in Shaping Health and Social Care Services*, Community Care Needs Assessment Project (CCNAP) (available from http://www.ccnap.org.uk) (accessed 7 March 2005).

Department of Health (2001) *Research Governance Framework for Health and Social Care*, London: DoH.

Hart, R. (1992) *Children's Participation: From Tokenism to Citizenship*, Innocenti Essays no. 4, Florence, Italy: UNICEF.

Redfern, M. (2001) *The Report of the Royal Liverpool Children's Inquiry*, London: The Stationery Office.

Rose, D. (2001) *User's Voices*, London: Sainsbury Centre for Mental Health.

Scott, J. (2003) *A Fair Day's Pay*, London: Mental Health Foundation.

Steel, R. (2003) *A Guide to Paying Members of the Public who are Actively Involved in Research*, 2nd edn, Eastleigh, Hampshire: INVOLVE.

Woodward, N. and Matthews, Z. (2000) 'Users as researchers: issues arising from a health service research project', in Y. Carter, S. Shaw and C. Thomas (eds) *Patient Participation and Ethical Considerations: Master Classes in Primary Care Research no. 5*, London: Royal College of General Practitioners.

Young Disabled People's Group (1996) *Resource Sheet 1*, Manchester: Greater Manchester Coalition of Disabled People.

Further reading

Barnes, C., Mercer, G. and Morgan, H. (1997) *Doing Disability Research*, Leeds: Disability Press (currently out of print but available http://www.leeds.ac.uk/disability-studies/archiveuk/) (accessed 7 March 2005).

Barnes, M. (1995) 'Research partnerships: working with groups', in G. Wilson (ed.) *Community Care: Asking the Users*, London: Chapman and Hall.

Baxter, L., Thorne, L. and Mitchell, A. (2001) *Small Voices, Big Noises: Lay Involvement in Health Research – Lessons from Other Fields*, Report by Folk.Us for Consumers in NHS Research, Exeter, Devon: Washington Singer Press.

Beresford, P. and Croft, S. (1993) *Citizen Involvement: A Practical Guide for Change*, London: Macmillan.

Butt, J., Box, L. and Lynn-Cook, S. (1999) *Respect: Learning Materials for Social Care Staff Working with Black and Minority Ethnic Older People*, London: Race Equality Unit, Home Office.

Campbell, J. and Oliver, M. (1996) *Disability Politics: Understanding our Past, Changing our Future*, London: Macmillan.

Carter, T. and Beresford, P. (2000) *Age and Change: Models of Involvement for Older People*, York: Joseph Rowntree Foundation.

Carter, Y., Shaw, S. and Thomas, C. (eds) (2001) *Patient Participation and Ethical Considerations: Master Classes in Primary Care Research no. 5*, London: Royal College of General Practitioners.

Kirby, P. (1999) *Involving Young Researchers: How to Enable Young People to Design and Conduct Research*, York: Joseph Rowntree Foundation.

Morris, J. (1998) *Don't Leave Us Out: Involving Disabled Children and Young People with Communication Impairments*, York: Joseph Rowntree Foundation.

Truman, C., Mertens, D. and Humphries, B. (eds) *Research and Inequality*, London: UCL Press.

Ward, L. (1997) *Seen and Heard: Involving Disabled Children and Young People in Research Projects*, York: Joseph Rowntree Foundation.

Wilkinson, H. (ed.) (2002) *The Perspectives of People with Dementia*, London: Jessica Kingsley.

Chapter 3

Supporting people with learning difficulties to do their own research

Val Williams and Mouse England

Some different inclusive research projects

> In the 'Journey to Independence' project, we have done all the research. We are people with learning difficulties, and the research is about how we think and see and understand. Other people who don't have a learning difficulty wouldn't be able to do it . . . some people may think that people with learning difficulties cannot be researchers, but we know that we can do it. In a lot of research, we are the exhibits. But now we are not just part of the picture – we are the artists of our lives.
>
> (Gramlich et al. 2002: 120)

This is how the Swindon People First research team conclude their report on a 30-month research project into direct payments support. The project, called 'Journey to Independence', employed three people with learning difficulties who worked in a team of researchers and supporters. One of us (Val) was their main research supporter. However, as employees of their own organization, run by people with learning difficulties, the team worked on a project that came directly from the interests of disabled people. In many ways, therefore, their project fulfilled the criteria given by Oliver (1992) for 'emancipatory research'.

There is a whole range of useful ways in which people with learning difficulties participate in research. Richardson (2000), for instance, describes a process whereby participants (the research 'subjects') are involved in checking out analysis and meanings with the researcher. Ward and Simons (1998) review the different modes of involvement, and Baxter et al. (2001) describe a scoping study of ways in which users, including people with learning difficulties, have been involved in social care and other research. Another example, with which we are familiar, is the 'Plain Facts' model (Townsley and Gyde 1997), where a person with learning difficulties is employed as part of a team, to make information about research accessible to other people with learning difficulties. This person's job is very well defined by the project he is working on, and involves checking text and pictures, commenting on them, preparing copy for publication, and helping to produce tapes.

There are still debates over whether 'emancipatory' research is possible where people with learning difficulties are concerned, because of their need for support. Working with non-disabled allies is often seen as a watering-down of true 'emancipatory research', although authors do sometimes recognize that it can be a step on the road towards emancipatory research (Zarb 1992). To cover this wide range of modes of involvement, Walmsley (2001) coined the term 'inclusive research', which describes well the ethos and background of this type of project. It is also a term that avoids the assumptions implicit in 'emancipatory' or 'participatory', and so seems a useful term to use in this chapter.

People with learning difficulties taking the lead

The usual practice in all the projects we describe in this chapter is for people with learning difficulties to be authors in their own right. In the present case, however, the focus is on how they get support. That is why Val Williams, as a research supporter and adviser, is the main author here. However, we will draw on many publications (formal and informal) from colleagues who have learning difficulties (Gramlich et al. 2002; Palmer et al. 1999). In addition, a member of the Bristol Self-Advocacy Research Group, Mouse England, has discussed a summary of the main points in this chapter, and her contributions are included in a contrasting font. Here, to start with, are her views on doing research and on the role of the supporter.

> How do we, as self-advocates, manage to do research? It depends on what research we are doing. We need support to do it, but we can take the challenge. Support is important. I like to have back-up, because if we are stuck we should always have some-one there to help us. Everyone's different, it's according to what you need. When we get support, does this mean we are not taking the lead?
>
> I think we are taking the lead for ourselves when we do research. We can get sup-port and take the lead. People may think we don't understand and we haven't got the guts to do it, but we say: 'Hang on. We need your support. We'll take the lead, and perhaps you can learn it from us.'

The role of the research supporter

In inclusive research, the work carried out by the adviser or supporter is of critical importance to many authors:

> If people with learning difficulties need non-disabled allies in the research process in order to convey their experiences in a way which is acceptable to the research community and its gatekeepers, how can the integrity of their accounts be maintained?
>
> (Chappell 2000: 41)

A non-disabled researcher who supports research is, in many ways, in a position parallel to that of supporters within the self-advocacy movement. Although People First and other such organizations are run directly by people with learning difficulties, they do nearly always have considerable support (Dowson and Whittaker 1993; Goodley 1997). The question is, can people with learning difficulties both have support and remain in control?

In practice, one of the main dilemmas faced by research supporters is the question of skills learning. While it may be true that all novice researchers need to learn, and indeed that access to learning should be considered a right for all, that very process of learning can paradoxically be disempowering for the learner (Swain 1995). In 'Journey to Independence', the research team felt that taking control of the process was an essential part of taking control of research. Thus, a central and guiding principle throughout the 'Journey to Independence' project was to ensure that the self-advocate researchers had access to the skills and resources they needed for research, while also supporting their ownership of and power over the whole project. To quote their report once more:

> Direct payments is about controlling our own lives!
> Self advocacy is about controlling our own lives
> Our research is about controlling our own research!
> That's why it all fits together.
> (Gramlich et al. 2002: 16)

Researchers with learning difficulties in action

To take a closer look at the work of researchers with learning difficulties, together with their research supporter, we are going to present some data from a different research project called 'Finding Out'. This same project is described by the research team in Palmer et al. (1999) and in Williams (1999) and is analysed in some depth in Williams (2002). The data and the observations made in this chapter are based on Williams (2002), to which readers are referred for a tighter and close-grained analysis.

'Finding Out' was quite a small project, in terms of its funding and status; the main players were four people who had the label of 'learning difficulty' and who decided to start their own research group. In the extracts below, they are given the names of Mark, Angela, Ian and Harry. They planned and carried out a short project, in which they wrote their own research questions, and fixed up group interviews with six other self-advocacy groups. Not only were the group interviews recorded, but also we kept the tape recorder on for much of the time during our preparation sessions.

Val Williams was a volunteer supporter for the group, having known three of the members previously through college courses and a new project called 'Europe People First'. At the time the Research Group started, we had started to hold sessions in the local People First offices, and two local supporters also had some involvement. This was how group members afterwards wrote about their ownership of the group:

> All the work is done by us. This gives us power, as researchers and as self-advocates in a way. But we also have to take responsibility. For instance, we are in charge of trying to get money for our group, and managing the money ourselves. It is a bit nerve-wracking, how to budget it, and we do get a bit of support with this. But it is our responsibility.
> (Palmer and Turner 1998: 12)

Clearly, a quotation such as that comes from a published document, and as such it is an important way of hearing the voices of people with learning difficulties. However, we all choose carefully the words in which we want our messages to be presented to a general readership, and people with learning difficulties are no different. In order to get closer to what actually happened, we will now look at some of the things we said, which were tape-recorded during our group sessions.

Who's going to post the letter?

The following scene took place as part of a session in which we were planning our research project, and organizing some of the research visits we were to make. Ian had been typing out a letter to one of the groups we were visiting, and had it ready in an envelope. Angela and the others were sitting round a table and waiting for Ian to join them for some group discussion.

Scene 1

1	*Val:*	Right so come on then Ian do you want to come and join us?
2	*Angela:*	Come on Mr Bolton.
3	*Ian:*	Yeah
4	*Val:*	Mr Bolton (*Ian walks over to join other members round table*)
5	*Ian:*	Oh, I'll leave the letter with you.
6	*Val:*	Thank you, well done doing that.
7	*Mark:*	He shouldn't (*whispering*)
8	*Angela:*	Yeah cos he might – he might forget to post it (*pause*)
9	*Ian:*	I'll post it, but I can't find (. . .)
10	*Angela:*	Give it to Val and she'll post it. It'll never – never get posted.

First, here are Mouse England's comments on this extract:

> One person in this group was writing a letter. But he didn't want to post it. I think he should do it for himself, otherwise he's just relying on someone else to do it for him. He's not showing people what he can do. Maybe he needs someone to nudge him to do things for himself.

What is happening in this brief exchange? First, the supporter gives an invitation (or even an instruction?) to Ian to come and join the group. It is the supporter who takes some responsibility for the design of the session, as well as the talk. Val asks Ian to leave the task he had been doing (printing out a letter) and to join the others. The implication is that we have something important to do, which warrants the full attention of all members. In coming to join the group, however, Ian decides to give Val the letter he has just printed, saying: 'Oh, I'll leave the letter with you'. By doing this, he is saying he is not going to follow through his task, and post the letter, but is entrusting it to the supporter. Why does this become an issue? Both Mark and Angela immediately disagree over who should post the letter:

7	*Mark:*	He shouldn't (*whispering*)
8	*Angela:*	Yeah cos he might – he might forget to post it (*pause*)

This exchange draws on shared understandings about the process in which we are engaged. If members are really in charge of this group, then they ought to be responsible enough to do their own work in organizing the group. It is their business and not the supporter's. However, Ian's comment, as interpreted by Angela, implies that he cannot even be trusted to post a letter. This brief exchange therefore signals an important issue in the group's progressive ownership of the business of research, which as it turns out will also be the main topic for our group discussion. Immediately after Ian joins the group, there is some talk about the minutes from the previous meeting. During that meeting, members had suggested things they would like to do in the research group (such as 'do some more visits' and 'write a book').

The supporter uses the authority of the written minutes to remind group members of the things they had decided they wanted to do. This strategy is even stronger than a memory jogger. The supporter not only reminds them of what they said before, but also encourages them to take responsibility for what they intend to do in the group. The implication of all these planned actions is that the research group is *theirs*: it belongs to them and exists only because of their plans. They need to take control of it. As Mouse comments:

> A supporter may say to me, 'If you want to read through the notes, then if there's something you want to change, you can change it.' It's good to have notes, but we should have a read, and change it if we want.

A few lines further on in the talk, this is precisely what happens – although in a rather unpredictable way. Mark brings up the subject of someone who has not attended the group recently:

Scene 2

29	*Mark:*	Well this thing about Judy
30	*Val:*	Yes?
31	*Mark:*	mm I did tell her
32	*Val:*	Oh thank you
33	*Mark:*	But I don't think – she may . . . I was going to get back to you
34		actually about Judy, she said she would like to come (.) on
35		Fridays, but I don't know what's happened to her today.
36	*Val:*	Perhaps – do you think I need to get in touch with her as well?

Mouse thinks it is important that Mark does take the lead in following up a missing group member:

> There's two ways of doing it. Either you can get a supporter to follow up, or you can do it yourself. That gives you the confidence. It'd be bad for the group if someone doesn't come, so it's up to us to find out why.

Mark not only gives a picture of himself as being active, in chasing up a missing group member, but also he assumes the right to judge both of her motives and the reasons for her absence. Mark takes on this role so effectively that the supporter asks his permission to share responsibility for group attendance: 'Perhaps – do you think

I need to get in touch with her as well?' (36), and goes on to effectively apologize for her non-action in this matter. The conversation at this point is in Mark's hands.

Doing interviewing

The scene we looked at above took place during a private group session; these were essentially occasions for preparation and learning. This was not of course all that happened in that project. The data collection consisted of group members visiting other groups to ask their research questions, and they conducted what became in essence 'focus groups' or group interviews. The supporter's role in those interviews was very much to stand back, and to let them make the running, and some of this was achieved by quite small effects. For instance, it was important for group members to:

* enter the room first
* take responsibility for introductions
* tell people what we were doing
* set up the tape recorder and ask for permission.

In the lives of people with learning difficulties, all of these things are frequently the responsibility of staff. In the context of our research, though, it was important that group members took responsibility themselves. This got them started off on a totally different footing with the interview, and helped them to be in charge of the flow of conversation. The supporter's role became minimal. The following extract is taken from the very first of the research visits, when Mark was starting out on the first of the questions they had planned to ask, which was about labelling. John and Darren are members of the group they were visiting.

Scene 3 (during a group interview)

81	*Mark:*	We're going to ask (um) yourself – what you think of the questions
82		we thought. The first one is, what do you think about people being
83		labelled. That's to – that to all of you . . .
		(*Mark looks round at everyone with a smile, and sweeps his hand round in a gesture.*)
84	*John:*	Well –
85	*Darren:*	What – sorry (. . .) you go.
86	*John:*	In what sort of way? Labelled in what sort of way?
87	*Mark:*	er – what do you think about people being labelled, being, like being –
88		umm like – like with a learning difficulty
89	*William:*	like – like – like us you mean?

Line 86 signalled a sticky moment for the group, and especially for Mark. This was the very first time that a particularly sensitive question was being posed, about labelling, and he had been challenged to explain himself. The video we made shows how he turned immediately to the supporter, with an expression that clearly said 'Help!' However, the supporter managed to support him simply by nodding and smiling, and he turned back to the original question, reading it out again. He then, however, added on the telling phrase 'with a learning difficulty', which led William to ask 'like us you mean?' This was precisely what Mark had been trying to avoid, as he and the group members had planned not to use the words 'learning difficulty' so as not to compromise or insult people they spoke with. During our original discussion on this issue, they had been helped to think through what they wanted to ask. However, during the interview itself, there was no intervention from the supporter. This is what Mouse had to say about Scene 3:

> It was important for one of our group to ask his own questions. It encourages him to be confident. Mostly, I can get the words out of my mouth alright. If I'm stuck, I would want support. It's according to how people are at the time. The supporter has got to judge how to help.

Even when researchers with learning difficulties clearly are getting into some deep waters, silence can be extremely important. Non-intervention signalled that they were indeed responsible and in charge of the situation. Eventually, as the analysis of this extended extract shows, they did manage to reach a position of meaningful understanding with each other, and the response to this first question was framed by one of the interviewees as:

104 *John:*   I think it's a bit of a cruel one, don't you, because it doesn't – it
105   does – it makes – it makes the people feel – it makes their problem
106   worse, the learning difficulty. It doesn't break down the
107   barriers/ it makes it – makes it bigger, doesn't it?

Mark, as the main interviewer at this point, accepts that response as something he can identify with, and so gives positive feedback to John.

108 *Mark:*   Yeah, it makes it – it affects a lot of people with a disability.
109   We found that in the group ourselves.

Becoming researchers

As a contrast to the extracts given above, we will now focus on a session in which we are reflecting on our research activities. This session came slightly later in the project, after the main set of group interview visits, when our aim was to produce material that we could use in writing about members' experience of doing research. We were engaged in recalling the interviews, to find out what we wanted to say about them and how members felt about their experiences. In order to do this, however, it was necessary first to establish what we were talking about.

Scene 4 (behind the scenes)

1   *Val:*   So, really you – you've – you can look back and see all the different
2   places you've been to –
3   *Ian:*   Oh yeah
4   *Angela:* You know I – I've got all the photographs in my photograph album

```
 5            at home . . .
 6  Val:      yeah
 7  Angela:   and I take it up the Shrubbery and show it to people . . .
 8  Val:      mm
 9  Angela:   And I'm quite proud of what I did . . . and I take it home at – at
10            Christmas and I went up and show it to Uncle Rob and Jenny . . . and his
11            girlfriend . . . and it's quite – it's quite – you feel quite really important.
12            I spoke to – I showed it to Tony today – he's my boss. 'Oh
13            you do do a lot then Angela', . . . and he was quite – he was
14            quite impressed with what I do.
```

This extract has been considerably cleaned up, with 'mms' and 'yeah' remarks mostly deleted. Some of Angela's false starts or repeats have also been deleted, so that it reads more easily. However, it can be appreciated that the research group members, especially Angela, are quite active in the conversation here. The supporter starts the ball rolling with 'you can look back and see all the different places you've been to' (1–2). Instead of simply referring to the research interviews or visits, she directs their attention to the locations, 'the places you've been to', which has the effect of making things more concrete.

Angela then takes over with her story, which starts at line 9. She takes up the theme of locations, to introduce the subject of her photos of our visits. More than that, she tells about how she has shown other people those photos: at home, the Shrubbery (a day centre) and at Uncle Rob's. The photographs perform a link role between the *places* we have visited and the *places* where they are shown to other people. Angela has picked up the general purpose of 'let's look back at what we have done', and helps us all to focus on those visits through talking about her photos. This was entirely her own choice of conversation; the photos, in fact, were not even present in the room.

At the end of this piece, she describes how she showed her photo album to her 'boss', and reports his reaction to it. Throughout, she uses words like 'impressed', 'proud', 'important'; Angela is particularly proud of being a researcher, especially in a context where she would normally be the client at the day centre, someone who is not expected to do something important like research.

The conversation between us goes on as follows:

Scene 5

```
15  Val:      Right, cause you know you . . . you can now say –
16  Angela:   Achieved a lot!
17  Val:      When you say something – carry on
18  Angela:   I have achieved a lot
19  Val:      mm hm
20  Angela:   Too much!
21  Val:      (laughter) and you've got a view of what other people think
22            outside of Norton now
23  Ian:      yeah
24  Harry:    yeah
25  Val:      which (.) makes it much more important.
```

The initial aim was to focus on the research visits, but Angela has moved on to talk about the *effect* of research on her own life. The supporter then builds on the scenario Angela has painted, by suggesting that she can 'say something' about her work, literally filling in a script between Angela and her boss. This script writing enables the talk to move very neatly back to the whole idea of what research is, the nature of their achievement. Not only do they have something to say in their own right but also, as researchers, they can report on what other people say:

> and you've got a view of what *other* people think outside of Norton now . . . which makes it much more important.

We are building up ideas together here, about the importance of what they have done. Support work like this simply builds on what people want to talk about, and as the team becomes more confident and more experienced, the supporter can step back. Ultimately, the goal is to become redundant, and to hand over as much as possible of the research process to the researchers with learning difficulties.

Conclusion: having a voice in developing research

It is hoped that this chapter has helped to throw light on the kind of activity that happens within some inclusive projects. However, the field of inclusive research with people with learning difficulties is very varied and rich, and there are probably as many different ways of working together as there are researchers and projects.

If we are concerned to include people with learning difficulties as researchers, it would make good sense to include them in the debates about the research process. In general, it is probably fair to say that the non-disabled researcher's perspective still dominates those debates and that literature. Researchers with learning difficulties have though sometimes written about the process in which they have engaged, and this chapter has drawn on much of this material. Some exciting initiatives are happening at present, and will hopefully help to swing the pendulum towards the voices of people with learning difficulties themselves who are involved in research. The UK Department of Health research initiative for 'Valuing People' has employed a group of leading self-advocates to act as monitors for the research projects funded under 'Valuing People' (Department of Health 2001). This group is making visits to each of the research projects to talk with people with learning difficulties there about their *own* perspectives on being involved in research.

The supporter will, for the foreseeable future, have some role to play in this process, and it is important that we work towards getting it right. By enabling people with learning difficulties to think for themselves, be active researchers, and develop their own knowledge base, it is hoped that they and their organizations will take a greater share in the future agenda of research. They need to decide for themselves what is important to research, what style of research they want to engage in, and what they get out of it. Research can be an exciting and powerful tool for change.

This is what Mouse England thinks is important for the future:

It comes back to projects. It's according to the subject they want to do. People say we're not powerful, but we are. I'd say we were just experts about our own future. It goes back to training – people with learning difficulties need good training to be researchers. People with learning difficulties can do things by themselves, or they can join a People First group, or they can work together with people who have done research before. Doing research is exciting, and it's something different.

We will leave the last words to members of the 'Finding Out' group, taken from one of our tapes:

Mark: I don't think you're going to get as much information from an MP [Member of Parliament] than you are from a researcher . . .
Val: Who has got the most power then?
Mark: People with learning difficulties.

References

Baxter, L., Thorne, L. and Mitchell, A. (2001) *Small Voices, Big Noises: Lay Involvement in Health Research – Lessons from Other Fields*, Report by Folk.Us for Consumers in NHS Research, Exeter, Devon: Washington Singer Press.

Chappell, A. (2000) 'Emergence of participatory methodology in learning difficulty research: understanding the context', *British Journal of Learning Disabilities*, 28: 38–43.

Department of Health (2001) *Valuing People: A New Strategy for Learning Disability for the 21st Century*, London: DoH.

Dowson, S. and Whittaker, A. (1993) *On One Side: The role of the Advisor in Supporting People with Learning Difficulties in Self Advocacy Groups*, London: Values Into Action.

Goodley, D. (1997) 'Locating self-advocacy in models of disability: understanding disability in the support of self-advocates with learning difficulties', *Disability and Society*, 12 (3): 367–79.

Gramlich, S., McBride, G., Snelham, N. and Myers, B. with Williams, V. and Simons, K. (2002) *Journey to Independence: What Self-advocates Tell us about Direct Payments*, Kidderminster: British Institute of Learning Disabilities (BILD).

Oliver, M. (1992) 'Changing the social relations of research production?', *Disability, Handicap and Society*, 7 (2): 101–14.

Palmer, N. and Turner, F. (1998) 'Self advocacy: doing our own research', *Royal College of Speech and Language Therapy Bulletin*, August: 12–13.

Palmer, N., Peacock, C., Turner, F. and Vasey, B. (1999) 'Telling people what you think', In J. Swain and S. French (eds) *Therapy and Learning Difficulties: Advocacy, Participation and Partnership*, Oxford: Butterworth-Heinemann.

Richardson, M. (2000) 'How we live: participatory research with six people with learning difficulties', *Journal of Advanced Nursing*, 32 (6): 1383–95.

Swain, J. (1995) 'Constructing participatory research: in principle and in practice', in P. Clough and L. Barton (eds) *Making Difficulties: Research and the Construction of SEN*, London: Paul Chapman.

Townsley, R. and Gyde, K. (1997) *Plain Facts*, York: Joseph Rowntree Foundation.

Walmsley, J. (2001) 'Normalisation, emancipatory research and inclusive research in Learning Disability', *Disability and Society*, 16 (2): 187–205.

Ward, L. and Simons, K. (1998) 'Practising partnership: involving people with learning difficulties in research', *British Journal of Learning Disabilities*, 26: 128–31.

Williams, V. (1999) 'Researching together', *British Journal of Learning Disabilities*, 27: 48–51.

Williams, V. (2002) 'Being researchers with the label of learning difficulty: an analysis of talk in a project carried out by a self-advocacy research group', unpublished PhD thesis, Open University, Milton Keynes.

Zarb, G. (1992) 'On the road to Damascus: first steps towards changing the social relations of research production', *Disability, Handicap and Society*, 7: 125–38.

Chapter 4

A hard fight

The involvement of mental health service users in research

A User Focus Monitoring Group

Introduction

We are a group of mental health service users who came together following an approach by the local health group (LHG). This is our story, of how we perceived the research project we were requested to undertake. The Trust had received funding from the LHG. This funding was used to establish a research-based project working in conjunction with the local university looking at acute psychiatric services offered by the local Trust. Initially the Sainsbury's Foundation for Mental Health was involved. This was the first time the Sainsbury's Foundation had done this type of research in Wales although they had done similar research many times before in England.

Setting up process

Adverts went out for two part-time co-ordinator posts. Service users were involved in the shortlisting and interviews. A mental health service user was employed to co-ordinate the project. He contacted many mental health groups and agencies and a meeting was set up between the service users and representatives from the Sainsbury's Foundation for Mental Health. At this meeting, we were told that we were going to be supplied with a computer, which at the end of the project would be given to the group of service users who would undertake the research. It was to be used for any future projects. This meeting was very successful; we were given a lot of information and offered a lot of support. We came away feeling very positive and enthusiastic about the project.

Following this, another meeting was set up between service users and the voluntary sector. This meeting was facilitated by the university. At the outset of this meeting, we were unsure of its purpose. During the course of the meeting, we felt that the agenda had already been discussed. It appeared that the voluntary sector along with the university had decided how the project should be run. It soon became apparent that the non-service users there wanted to run the show. Many of us felt that we were just being used to rubber stamp the process and that we were not true partners in the project. We felt our input was not really wanted. It was a very demoralizing experience as we were regarded as ill and incapable.

The voluntary sector and the university put great pressure on the service users to have all the interviews taped. The service users felt this to be a bad idea, but the pressure was still applied. A service user telephoned the Sainsbury's Foundation for Mental Health about taping the interviews. They were fully supportive of the service user group, as they had found in the past that tape-recording brought zero response. Things got so heated that, at one stage, the Mind representative (who was very supportive) decided to take the non-service users out of the room. This allowed the service users to make decisions as to who should be involved in the process. The newly appointed co-ordinator was strongly supportive of the service users but, even at this early stage, it was obvious that his job was under threat if he did not support the university standpoint. The stance taken by the university and voluntary sector was aggressive and negative. This resulted in some service users having to leave the meeting. Some found the experience so distressing that they never returned. One person became so ill they were later hospitalized. Some rejoined the group. One service user ended up self-harming:

> The pressure in the room was so much; so much hostility and I felt we were being used as tokens, they had their own agenda. I felt I was nothing I just had to know I was a human being.

However, despite all of this, a group of service users was formed and came to be known as the User Focus Monitoring (UFM) group.

Relationship with the university

From the start, we were keen to work with the university as we felt this would give our work greater credibility. We were led to believe that we would receive good training and support. However, this did not materialize. We were given half a day's training, which later proved to be totally inadequate for this type of research. Throughout the whole of the project, the relationship was strained. We were told that the money we needed to run the project would be available from the university. At times, it was difficult to get the money. Even when we got to the right department, with the right forms, we would be told that there was no money there for us. This happened to several people many times.

Post-interview support in this type of project is of great importance – interviews can be very distressing to the interviewer and interviewee. Some interviewers felt that they had been put in very threatening situations. The arrangement was that we would ring the university and that support would be available. We would ring the university, but sometimes were unable to speak to anyone, other times we would get through but there was no support forthcoming.

Finances

From the beginning, the group was told that money was short, but that it would be possible to pay some expenses and to give people an interview fee. During the setting up of the project, it was necessary for the group to meet on a regular basis. We provided our own tea etc., and travelling expenses were not claimed because of the hassle involved in doing so. We were encouraged to look around for the cheapest venue in which to hold the meetings. We ended up in some pretty grim places. Even so, we managed to do the work necessary to get the project underway. While we were shopping around for the cheapest church hall, members of the statutory and non-statutory bodies, who were indirectly involved, had an all expenses paid weekend in London. The cost of this was taken from the UFM budget. These anomalies highlight the great divide between service users and service providers. This certainly did nothing for the self-esteem of the service users.

Writing the questionnaires

A period of twelve weeks was spent developing the questionnaire. During this time, the group felt that they were being put under enormous pressure from outside agencies. For the service users to remain in charge of the process, the whole group had to be very strong and determined. Early on in the question writing, the group was informed that the Sainsbury's Foundation was no longer involved in the service user part of the project. Some of the service users had in the past worked with a member of the university from a different department. They had found working with this person was a very positive experience and felt that they had learnt a lot from the exercise. When the UFM group said they would like to contact him to ask for advice about the questions, the university was very adamant that that no contact should be made.

Some of the questions we were asked to put in weren't even relevant. Some were put in to keep them happy. All the questions had to be written up and the format of the questionnaire developed. The group undertook this work. A service user took the questions home and used their own computer for the task. The computer that had been purchased was based at the university but the group did not have access to it. Many times the questionnaire was altered and reprinted. Neither paper nor ink was supplied, and it was the service users who bore the cost of this themselves.

Eventually the process of compiling the questionnaires was completed. It consisted of 89 quantitative and qualitative questions. To have a feel for the completed questionnaires, we spent some time working in pairs role-playing. This caused a number of problems for many people, the most obvious problem being that each interview was going to take a long time to complete. The process of role-play itself evoked painful memories for many people. As a result, some members decided not to be involved in the actual interview process as it would be far too emotional and difficult for them. Luckily, they choose to remain involved with the group but not in the capacity of interviewers. The members who were left feeling distressed after these sessions looked to the university for support. Unfortunately, none was forthcoming.

During this period, the co-ordinator not only had personal pressure in his life, but also had pressure from the university to make us comply with their wishes. At times, the co-ordinator's job became almost impossible as he was supposed to arbitrate between the group, the university and other agencies involved. There were times when this became so difficult that this adversely affected the co-ordinator's health. We feared for the continuation of the project. The co-ordinator was unwell and unable to be supportive to the group. He started to turn against some members of the UFM group. The group felt that there was no actual support available for him. It was felt that the co-ordinator's job was on the line if he supported us. The inadequacy of the training we had been given again showed itself. One of the members of the group was obviously unwell throughout the process. As a group, we just continued with the project. Really, we should have been taught how to handle the situation. This support should have come from the university, via the co-ordinator. However, the co-ordinator was unwell at times himself, and the university appeared to be unable to provide the support that both the co-ordinator and the group needed.

Doing the interviews

To ensure random selection and maintain patient confidentiality, it was decided by the group that the first 100 patients discharged from the acute psychiatric services under study after a certain date would be sent letters asking them to take part in the research. We needed 30 ex-patients. Of the first 100 letters sent out, not enough service users replied. So a further 100 letters were also sent to the next 100 patients discharged. This time, by including both mail shots, we had the amount of responses needed to complete the research. The hospital initially sent out the letters giving the university as the contact for any replies. The group was provided with a list of names and contact details, which was shared among the group. The group split into pairs to do the interviewing, one to ask the questions and one to write the report. Due to confidentiality, nothing was known about the interviewees before hand. No vetting was undertaken as to their suitability or mental health at that time. Many of the interviews took place in the client's own homes, so placing the interviewers in extremely vulnerable situations. No training had been giving in how to deal with difficult situations. We were unaware of even basic techniques like sitting near the door! Nor were we made aware of how to ensure our own safety while doing the interviews, or how to deal with volatile or dangerous situations that may arise.

The half-day's training we received in no way prepared us for the task. It consisted of basic interview techniques. These interviews were far from basic. The interviews themselves could last for up to an hour or more and became quite intense. We had vastly differing experiences of the actual interviews. Some interviews went smoothly. Some people we interviewed found it a relief to be able, at last, to talk to someone about their experiences. They felt the experience was unique to themselves and that no one else was aware of what it had been like to be a patient there. It was good for them to realize that they weren't on their own. These interviews initially were easy to cope with, but after interviewing a few like this, it left some interviewers distressed. Some of the interviewers had been patients at the hospital and it just brought back to them the feelings associated with their own experience of being a patient there. Some of the interviewers were shocked and numbed with the realization that it was not the occasional patient but so many patients who had such a bad experience while being inpatients.

Other interviews, however, were much harder to cope with. Interviewers came out feeling very vulnerable. Some of the people they had interviewed were clearly still very unwell, and having being given no training in what to do in these circumstances, it left some interviewers feeling very distressed. The system that was set up for debriefing failed. Many calls were made to the university for help or just to talk. Most of them were unanswered. Some people carried around the feelings and apprehension with them. The group ended downloading on each other. This did have an impact on some of the service users' mental health. While no one was admitted to hospital, it did affect some members of the group's mental state for months. A few interviewees became agitated. Again, we as interviewers had had no training on how to deal with these situations. The only advice given was 'get out fast', not *how* to get out fast or who to call for help if necessary. We were so lucky that none of us were physically hurt or found ourselves in very compromising situations. A number to ring afterwards is of no use, especially as, most of the time, no one was there to answer the phone. Often, no one in the university was aware of when the interviews took place; there was no way of checking if we were safe or not. The project co-ordinator lived a long way from the area where the study was being undertaken and, therefore, was not easily accessible for help or support.

The research report

On completion of all 30 interviews, it became obvious that the group was not going to be involved in the writing of the report. The report was being written at the university. While this was happening, the UFM group had to keep pushing to be informed of any progress, and to have any involvement in its contents. Eventually, the university agreed to bring a draft report to the UFM group and, at this stage, we were allowed minimal input and some alterations were agreed. We feel this was just another unnecessary difficult battle for the group. Actually doing the interviews had not been a very positive experience and everyone was shocked by the results. The group wanted a report that truthfully reflected our findings and not a report that was acceptable to the Trust.

In the final draft document, there were two reports. There were the findings from the UFM group and there was a separate report based upon research involving the hospital staff. Members of the UFM group did have sight of the final draft UFM report, which was kept at the university, but we were not given copies. The Trust had a copy of the draft document and asked that we did not say anything to anyone about our report. They wanted time to read the draft document and make decisions regarding the impact it would have once in the public domain. An intended launch date was given. However, this date came and went with no mention of a launch being made.

As time went on, the draft document was leaked to the press. The conclusions of the draft document caused a media frenzy. This resulted in excerpts from the draft document making front-page headlines in the local press. The story was then picked up by BBC Wales, making national news. The article in the media had not clarified that the draft report was only concerning the standards of care in the acute wards. This caused much distress for elderly patients, their carers and the hospital staff. The standard of care for the elderly people in the hospital is exemplary and was never in question. At meetings, members of the UFM group were made to feel very uncomfortable. Hints were made that it could only be service users that would do such a thing. Comments like 'don't table any confidential reports when service users are around as reports get leaked' were made. Although some members of the group may have felt like leaking the draft document, we still had not been given a copy of the staff report. Consequently, no one in the group could possibly have been responsible for the leaking of the documents. It was apparent that there was an appalling attitude to people with a mental health problem, insinuating that having a mental health problem renders people untrustworthy.

Due to all the media interest, one member of the group was inundated by visits from the press at home. It made life very difficult for this individual. A report into a local psychiatric hospital hits the headlines. It is ironic that the people who were asked on television to comment were people who had nothing to do with the report. They knew nothing about the hospital in question.

Conclusion

This chapter has concentrated on the collective experiences of the UFM group and the 'interviewers' during the process of the research project. To academics, the label 'research project' implies the collection of data. We believe that our findings were regarded in a very detached way. The collection of data and information is a means to an end. In order that change may occur, data was needed to prove or disprove the validity of the services provided on the acute psychiatric wards in the hospital. Yet, two years on, we still have strong concerns regarding the interviewees who gave their time to enable this research to happen. They freely discussed events that happened to them at a very distressing time in their lives. At no time during the project was any thought given to how *they* may feel about the process and how *they* would feel after been interviewed. Some interviewees had very traumatic experiences while in the hospital. Discussing these during the interviews brought back vivid memories and emotions for them. While it may have helped some of them to have a chance to talk about these things, there is no way of knowing how they coped during the following days. There was no support provided for the interviewees. We had no contact name or number to give to them should they need to talk to someone afterwards. How many of these people suffered for it afterwards? We don't know. No one visited them to see how these interviews affected them at the time or afterwards.

Looking back, would we have done it if we had known in advance what would have happened? The answer to this is a double-edged sword. Was this really worth the risk to the interviewers' state of health? Some members of the UFM group were taken seriously ill and even hospitalized due to the stress of the process. Others became unwell for an extended period of time. One member of the group became antagonistic due to the stress, resulting in a physical attack upon another member of the group. This highlights the lack of resources and support, which is essential to this type of work, being made available to the group. In addition, it is obvious, that if this kind of project should be undertaken in the future, then agencies such as the university should have training in how to work with service users.

The other edge to the sword is that because of the report, positive changes have taken place. Life for acute patients on the ward has significantly improved. Changes to working practices have been made. The physical ward environment has been upgraded in response to the recommendations within the report. Occupational therapists now work on the wards with the patients.

So looking back would we have done it? Yes, we would. As a group, we have gained knowledge, confidence and expertise. We have become stronger as individuals and as a group. We have learned to value ourselves. Consequently, the UFM group has stayed together and is now being commissioned to undertake further projects. Projects that we can say are truly user led.

Despite the negativity encountered throughout the process, the overall outcome is that the project has had an impact on the services provided in the acute wards. Positive changes, and changes that were asked for within the recommendations, have been implemented. The hospital has changed, but it still has a long way to go and 'the chips are still cold'.

Chapter 5

Translating health policy into research practice

Paula Hodgson and Krysia Canvin

Introduction

The aim of this chapter is to explore and critically appraise the recent moves towards consumer involvement in health research. The UK government has attempted to initiate cultural shifts in how health research is undertaken through policy documents that direct researchers to involve consumers in all aspects of the research process, such as *Patient and Public Involvement in the New NHS* (Department of Health (DoH) 1999a), *Research and Development for a First Class Service* (DoH 2000a) and *Research Governance Framework for Health and Social Care* (DoH 2002). This is reinforced by the requirement that Trusts holding NHS research and development funding have to provide evidence of involving consumers in their research activity as a condition of continued funding (DoH 2000a). The rhetoric of the 'consumer movement' within health care is unrelenting, politically expedient, and morally impervious. As such, the principle of consumer involvement in health research is resistant to criticism: it is appropriate that the recipients of health care should have a voice in policy and practice. However, we suggest that in practice this policy is fundamentally flawed, both theoretically and practically. We do not take a 'Luddite' stance towards consumer involvement in health research, but we do consider that its current construction (in the policy documents) is problematic and we illustrate our argument with case study examples from our work with consumers.

In this chapter, we argue that as currently conceptualized, health research and consumer involvement are incompatible due to a range of obstacles: from conceptualizing 'consumer involvement in health research' to actually 'involving' consumers in health research. We begin the chapter by reviewing the historical and political context of health research, and examining the dominance of the scientific method in health research and government policy. Second, we trace the events and political shifts that led to the emergence of consumers, arguing that consumer involvement has arisen out of a particular set of cultural circumstances and has been incorporated into health policy for politically expedient reasons with little acknowledgment of the epistemological challenge it poses. Third, we propose that in order to operationalize consumer involvement, 'health research' must be translated, and this may lead to the development of different models of health research that incorporate consumer knowledge. We conclude the chapter by discussing the implications of our analysis for consumer involvement in health research and proposing a way forward.

The historical and political context of consumer involvement in health research

The scientific method and dominant forms of knowledge in health research

Central to our analysis is the notion that consumers 'involved' in health research will be faced with language, discourses and practices that are alien to them; while conversely, there are health researchers who are steeped in methodological frameworks and models of health and illness that have developed over centuries of scientific inquiry and, as such, are taken-for-granted. For us, this tension is at the heart of what is problematic about consumer involvement in health research. To appreciate how the research world came to conceptualize 'health research' in its present form, and how this is inherently problematic for consumer involvement in health research, we will briefly trace the origins of the dominance of the scientific method and the biomedical model.

Health research, as an activity, is closely associated with the scientific method that has developed, and is undertaken within positivist and empirical frameworks that can be traced back to the Enlightenment. The Enlightenment is often viewed as the starting point for the 'birth' of science where observation and deduction were more clearly formalized with the concomitant notion that scientific knowledge is based on facts. The Enlightenment can be seen as a reaction to the authority of religion and the work of the philosopher Aristotle (Chalmers 1999).

A positivist approach includes a belief in the scientific method in order to study and reconstruct the social, political and economic domains to achieve social progress, and that human nature is fixed despite an ever-changing society. The work of the social sciences can be considered to be the observation of human nature and the construction of social laws that explain these constants. Broadly speaking, empiricists hold the view that all knowledge should be derived from ideas implanted in the mind by way of sense perception. Both empiricism and positivism share the common view that scientific knowledge, or 'facts', are arrived at through objective observation.

Key concepts of the scientific method emerged from the work of René Descartes (1596–1650) and Immanuel Kant (1724–1804) and include the autonomy of the human subject who is capable of acting in a conscious manner; the search for universal 'truths' that are achieved through associating the social and physical realities; the social and natural world are situated within a natural sciences model; and the gathering of systematic knowledge over time (May 1996). These scientific values underpin the notion and activity of health research 200 years on. Indeed, the colonization of the scientific method and its associated knowledge aided by the essential tools of the scientist, objectivity and reason, has dominated and transcended any other type of knowledge.

However, the history and sociology of scientific knowledge reveals that such scientific work is not as simple as this model suggests and science and its purported facts are not quite so certain (Bloor 1976; Latour and Woolgar 1986; Knorr-Cetina 1981; Gilbert and Mulkay 1984; Lynch 1998; Collins and Pinch 1993). For example, a scientist/researcher cannot assume that water will always boil at 100 degrees Celsius, as a number of variables, such as altitude and water purity, can interfere with outcomes.

The separation of the mind and the body through the work of Descartes underpins the biomedical model that dominates medical knowledge and practice. Combined, the scientific method and the biomedical model have pervaded health research and contributed to the construction of medical knowledge, and in turn, medical practice. For instance, a one-way model of communication in health information sheets derives from the dominant discourse of the biomedical framework rather than other forms of information and knowledge (Dixon-Woods 2001). In this way, lay beliefs and knowledge are sidelined with individuals having to make choices from information that is medically driven with all the connotations of power and compliance. Latterly, we have witnessed the advent of more complex and broader models of health and illness. The inclusion of psychological, sociological, and indeed, cultural factors in the development and treatment of illness has widened our understanding and management of illness (or the maintenance of health). However, the biomedical model persists in the form of the randomized controlled trial: hailed as the 'gold standard'.

The emergence of the 'consumer'

'Consumerism' is a cultural phenomenon that has emerged since World War II. The conception and implementation of the welfare state in Britain was a bold move to address the perceived 'five giants' – want, disease, ignorance, idleness and squalor (Beveridge 1942). The newly elected Labour government of 1945 implemented large-scale nationalization and created welfare institutions, such as the NHS, that would entitle its citizens to feel protected and to, at least notionally, be a part of a society that had universalism as a central tenet. However, as the economic prosperity of the United Kingdom started to grow under the influence of post-war policies, austerity was replaced by a desire for change, reflected in the social unrest of the 1960s. By the time of the 1973 oil crisis, the notion of the state being able to provide for all was severely diminished, and increasingly the welfare state was seen as a barrier to economic productivity (Mishra 1984).

Subsequently, the 1970s saw major reforms to the welfare state. In particular, the NHS underwent significant changes in its structure, with an emphasis on management and planning. Increasingly, it was acknowledged that patients were important and needed to be 'heard', and this was reflected in a number of government documents and party manifestos (Klein 1983). The Community Health Councils (CHCs), in particular, heralded the beginning of increased accountability beyond civil servants and health professionals: one-third of their membership was made up of nominees of voluntary organizations who represented patients' views (Klein and Lewis 1976). Such representation was nominal in the ability of the representatives to impact upon the running of health authorities, as the role of the CHCs was relatively passive.

The *Griffiths Report* (Griffiths 1983) included an acknowledgement of the need to understand service users' experiences and perceptions of health care. Furthermore, the Conservative governments of the 1980s moved towards consumer demands for health care, based upon individual needs. This move reflected broader reinterpretations of the welfare state; from universal and accessible state benefits, to reduced levels of commitment by the state to support its citizens. Indeed, following another review of health services in 1989 and the introduction of market principles (DoH 1989) such notions were at the forefront of change through the introduction of managed competition where service users were to pick the best service providers to fulfil their needs. Eventually leading to the publication of *The Patients' Charter* (DoH 1991). These changes have been continued by the New Labour government and the 'third way' (Giddens 1998).

Perhaps one of most salient indicators of the cultural changes that occurred during the 1980s is the language used by government agencies and in wider discourses: from patient, to service user and consumer. This language attempted to capture the renegotiated relationship between the state and its citizens, and health care providers and health care users. The notion of the consumer and its importance to reconceptualizing this relationship has been noted by other authors (Ewen 1976; McKendrick et al. 1982; Featherstone 1983; Miller 1987; Baudrillard 1988; Bauman 1987, 1988). The term 'consumerism' is derived from an economic model of a free market where consumers will purchase those services or goods that they want or meet their needs, and will determine the success or failure of the producers of goods. Additionally, there is a tacit assumption that the type and quality of services and goods will improve as consumers search out the best products. Thus, one of the central tenets of 'consumerism' is that power shifts from those who provide services to those who consume them.

In the context of the NHS, this model suggests that providers of health care, such as doctors, nurses and managers, should accommodate the demands of the consumer rather than providing health care based on professional interests. Concomitantly, this requirement to meet consumers' demands should diminish health care professionals' authority and help to develop a more equal (and satisfying) relationship between provider and user. However, this idealized relationship is flawed. First, the relationship between the user and producer is not based on equal power to control the encounter (Abercrombie 1994). Thus, the power imbalance in the relationship will continue to be reproduced, albeit in a different form. Second, the ability of the consumer to actualize this rhetoric requires both parties to be 'culturally drenched' (Featherstone 1991) in the same language and discourses. If the consumer is unable to display some form of agency in their exchange with the provider (through the use of particular language that exemplifies 'insider' knowledge) then there will be dissonance between the provider and the user. The voice of the consumer is often reduced to an artificial form of involvement, tokenism, or a failure to encompass the values associated with consumer involvement. Medicine and its practitioners have been extremely powerful (and successful) in retaining their knowledge and authority. Thus, in practice, the meaning of consumer representation and empowerment can be modified and translated by 'experts' who retain their power as the very structures and organizations that are asking for consumer input remains firmly within their grasp.

The concept of 'empowerment' is inextricably linked to ideas about consumers, consumers' rights and consumers' responsibilities. At the heart of this is the notion that consumers have rights and voices that must be heard and upheld. Consumer empowerment became a crucial activity within the NHS with numerous surveys undertaken on issues such as rationing and preferences for health care provision. However, the needs of consumers, as represented through surveys, could be met only when professional interests coincided with them: to articulate a need does not necessarily produce a response. Furthermore, consumer empowerment discourses led to the renegotiation of public health approaches to include the caveat that the consumer had to become more responsible for her/his health (Nettleton 1997). Thus, public health surveys encouraged individuals to reflect upon their own lifestyles in an attempt to uncover healthy and unhealthy behaviour (Ogden 1995) as well as asking consumers to record their needs from health care services.

Another catalyst in consumer involvement in health research was the government's desire to make the NHS more accountable to the public. This can be seen clearly in the publication of several key documents including *The New NHS: Modern and Dependable* (DoH 1997), *The Expert Patient* (DoH 2001a), *Research Governance Framework for Health and Social Care* (DoH 2002) and a series of *National Service Frameworks* for mental health (DoH 1999b), coronary heart disease (DoH 2000b) and older people (DoH 2001b) that signalled the arrival of a 'New NHS'. Central to these reforms were the introduction of 'clinical excellence' (to be measured using random-ized controlled trials), public accountability, the acknowledgement of the expertise of patients with chronic illness, and consumer involvement. These policies were precipi-tated by a series of adverse events (Nicholls et al. 2000) and subsequent inquiries. For example, research and clinical practices at the Alder Hey and Bristol hospitals were found to be unethical (the former involved the removal of organs and body tissues from dead children without parental consent, the latter involved higher than average mortality rates following paediatric surgery) (DoH 2000c, 2001c). The inquiries rec-ommended increased transparency and accountability in health research and clinical practice. Combined, these events transformed health research, especially the issue of informed consent. Guidelines now indicate that a signature on a consent form is no longer adequate for an individual to be involved in research: researchers must now ensure that the individual fully understands the research project. Additionally, informed consent must now be obtained for all research procedures, including those pertaining to the use of tissue samples (e.g. blood) held in storage, and non-invasive procedures (such as interviews) with NHS patients or staff (DoH 2001c).

To summarize, the notion of a 'consumer' arose out of a specific political context where individuals were transformed from patients, with all the connotations of pas-sivity, medical surveillance, and a biomedical model of health care, into active con-sumers choosing from health care options. The use of the term 'consumer' in health research assumes that an individual is similarly transformed into an active agent who will be able to make informed choices about involvement in health research.

We suggest that, against the backdrop of the 'scientific method', the UK govern-ment have merged concepts and principles from the consumer or user movement and participatory action research (PAR) (which we consider to be the, albeit distant, ori-gin of consumer involvement). Cornwall and Jewkes (1995: 1671) usefully describe participatory research or participatory action research as 'more of an attitude or approach than a series of techniques'. We argue that the attempt to integrate the com-peting models of PAR (commonly employed in anthropology, but less so in health research) and the scientific method is both theoretically and practically flawed. A number of assumptions underlie health research as we know it nowadays: that the 'truth' exists and can be uncovered through the use of experimental methods that prize objectivity and replicability as ways of assuring the validity and reliability of the findings. In contrast, PAR is a collaborative approach between researchers and par-ticipants that looks at the practical concerns of people in problematic situations and furthers the goals of social science simultaneously. Thus, there is a dual commitment in PAR to study a phenomenon and concurrently collaborate with members of the system in changing it in what is together regarded as a desirable result. Accomplishing such goals requires the active collaboration of researchers and participants, and thus, focuses on the importance of co-learning in the research process. One of the core tenets of PAR is that each individual's contributions are of equal significance in all aspects of the research process, such as the interpretation and analysis of data. Furthermore, PAR attempts to avoid the prior knowledge imbalance between researchers and participants as it allows for the different ways of 'seeing'.

On reflection, consumer involvement is subject to a continuing power imbalance between medical practitioners and individuals, and reliant on concurrence between the wants/needs of both sets of actors. Several assumptions underlie the policy: it is assumed that researchers wish to involve consumers, and that consumers wish to be involved, and it is assumed that researchers know how to involve consumers and con- sumers know how to get involved (or that they can get involved) (see Case Study 1). Most significantly, it assumes that there are groups of people who can be categorized as 'consumers' and fails to acknowledge the difficulties of defining 'involvement' (see Case Study 2). At present, consumer involvement merely maintains the status quo by appearing to attempt to incorporate competing perspectives, when it actually amounts to tokenism. It is within this problematic framework that researchers are expected to involve consumers, and consumers are expected to lead or conduct research. Ultimately, the involvement of consumers in health research requires the translation of these core concepts and values, and their adaptation to accommodate multiple kinds of knowledge.

Competing forms of knowledge: incorporating consumer knowledge

As noted above, the advent of the consumer within health care practices, and perti- nently for this chapter, consumer involvement in health care research, is situated in the context of increased accountability and transparency of the research process and increased acknowledgement of other forms of knowledge.

Sociological investigations of the public's understanding of scientific knowledge have been particularly fruitful in challenging the authority of science and the impor- tance of including other forms of knowledge. The 'public deficit model' as discussed in the Public Understanding of Science (PUS) literature focuses on the apparent gap between lay and 'expert' scientific or professional understanding. The notion of such a 'gap' assumes some form of deficiency on the part of the public and is said to lead to inappropriate behaviour such as non-compliance with medical advice, failure to abstain from risky behaviour, or not consulting doctors appropriately (Bury 1997; Good 1994; Irwin and Wynne 1996b). Furthermore, the public deficit model would also suggest that the public are ill informed and protest irrationally against legitimate scientific activities (Elston 1994). It also implies a more general inability of the public to play their part as informed citizens in democratic debate (Irwin and Wynne 1996b; Michael 1996). The 'solution' that is generally forwarded to overcome such a 'deficit' proposes an increase in the public's scientific or medical literacy, with an implicit assumption that science/medicine holds the high ground in its knowledge base.

Criticisms of the public deficit model do not generally contest that the general pub- lic falls short when measured by the standards of expert science/medicine (Wynne

1991, 1996; Williams and Popay 1994). But, there have been criticisms of the presumption that the universalist knowledge of 'expert' science is the appropriate standard, and that the greater the exposure the public have to such knowledge the greater the chance that a sceptical public will be converted towards accepting scientific claims. Critics also argue that greater attention has to be paid to the context of the public understanding of science and medicine: instead of the categorical distinctions between an undifferentiated lay understanding and an equally undifferentiated expert, the proposal is for a more relational view (Irwin and Wynne 1996b; Michael 1996). This would enable the local knowledge of workers, the experiential knowledge of people with chronic illness, the variable distribution of expert knowledge among health professions and the challenges posed by lay activities to expert science to be recognized (Wynne 1996; Grinyer 1995; Bury 1997; Collins et al. 1998; Epstein 1995; Indyk and Rier 1993). And, the complex mixture of lay trust and lay scepticism towards medicine/science could emerge (Williams and Calnan 1996).

Penetrating and translating the world of health research

Consumer involvement in health research policy fails to acknowledge that there has to be a degree of integration and assimilation for consumers to penetrate the world of health research (see Case Study 1). Individual researchers could be said to occupy a 'social world' (Strauss 1978) or 'community of practice' (Lave and Wenger 1991) where practices and discourses are commonly understood and involve relationships with other people who do similar things (Becker 1986; Clark and Fujimura 1992; Clark and Montini 1993). Membership is a complex process and can depend on how long they remain within a particular social world but can be learnt through a process of 'legitimate peripheral participation' (Lave and Wenger 1991). Crucially, we want to stress that, as with any type of work, there are high levels of 'insider' knowledge that are essential requisites of carrying out research. From familiarity with the research field to researching the current state of knowledge about a topic to conducting, analysing and interpreting the research – these are all run of the mill activities to a researcher. Health research involves blending specialist, technical knowledge or expertise with a range of strategies and methods that can appear, on the face of it, common sense. However, in health research, particular methodologies are employed to answer specific questions. The research process requires a host of actors (trained extensively in research methods and able to apply their expert knowledge), technologies (computers, software, university libraries), organizations (universities, the NHS, funding bodies, ethics committees) and financial resources (all research has a cost). Finding and assembling all of the complex components that need to be found, accessed and used is an intricate accomplishment that requires specialist training and some degree of acceptance by the research community, i.e. via peer review. The multifaceted nature of 'doing research' highlights another problematic aspect of consumer involvement policy: the assumption that consumers may be simply integrated into existing methods of research. The result has been the emergence in (research and clinical) practice of a competing notion of consumer involvement: that it is highly problematic and impractical. We suggest that neither is helpful in terms of moving the debate forward.

'Social worlds theory' is helpful in this respect, not only illuminating the problems of integrating consumers, but also indicating potential ways in which we can begin to address some of the issues. Researchers from different social worlds have common practices, such as the adoption of particular theories or methods (Fujimura 1986, 1988) that help to stabilize the research community's approaches to particular questions. The notion of stabilization is helpful when considering the translation of health research by and for consumers. For Latour (1987), stabilization occurs when scientists/researchers construct a transportable and standardized theory-method package (such as DNA technologies) and then transport this package into different social worlds. One of the benefits of a standardized package is to 'translate the interests' of many members of different social worlds (different laboratories, funding agencies and technology companies) to facilitate increased interaction among researchers and a more rapid development of research. To facilitate consumer involvement in this way, health researchers must construct (in conjunction with consumers) a transportable and standardized theory-method package to transport into the social world of the consumer. Attempts to do so far have included 'transferable lessons' and 'guides' on how to involve consumers (and for consumers on how to get involved) and have prioritized the conduct of technical processes (e.g. research question formulation, data collection) in their simplest form and are, as a result, theoretically and conceptually barren (see, for example, Hanley et al. 2003; Royle et al. 2001; Thorne et al. 2001).

Furthermore, to become part of a social world involves rules and practices within any given community and also involves encountering the objects involved in practices, including tools, texts and symbols (Bowker and Star 2000). For example, Michael Polanyi (1973) describes the changes in a medical student's perceptions of X-rays. Initially, the film has little meaning, but as the student is taught to interpret the depth and shape of shadows, the picture can reveal previously hidden representations of the body: the student can then start to medically interpret X-rays. Eventually such encounters can lead to a familiarity that within anthropology is considered to be the 'naturalization' of categories or objects (Schutz 1944) (see Case Study 2).

The application of 'social worlds theory' to consumer involvement alerts us to the potential effects of integrating consumers into the social world of health researchers. How can consumers become part of a research social world? What depth of knowledge do consumers need to be participants in health research? Do consumers have to have the same or equivalent knowledge as researchers? If consumers do not have the requisite technical expertise, must they be trained? And, if they receive such training, do they then become researchers and cease to be consumers? If consumers' lay expertise and (research) naivety are at the core of why their involvement might be valuable to health research, their integration into the social world of research seems to contradict, indeed disable this contribution as their conformity to the dominant discourse of health research pervades the way that they see the world.

One aspect of research and methodology that consumers could contribute without training is their expertise: their lay perceptions and experiences of health, illness and health research (see Case Study 2). While the incorporation of (or need for) user perspectives or input is apparent both in the policies, the literature and examples of consumer involvement, it has been substantially undermined in several ways. There has been a systematic failure to acknowledge the consumer perspective as a legitimate way of knowing: it is highly situated, individual knowledge that reflects cultural and experiential influences, and as such does not 'fit' comfortably within a scientific/medical arena. Inevitably, consumer/lay knowledge is often sidelined when it is pitted against a positivistic framework, as it is deemed irrelevant for the very reason that gives it strength, it is individualistic (Ong 1996). When scrutinizing the lay paradigm, a key issue arises: it is based within the individual narrative, and therefore highly variable. This individualistic basis represents both the strength, that is, the cultural subjectivity and depth of experience, and the weakness of lay knowledge, namely that penetrating the medico-scientific paradigm is done in a fragmented fashion, thus blunting the power of the alternative perspective. It is all too easy, therefore, to dismiss lay knowledge as ad hoc and irrelevant to medical science (Ong 1996).

There has also been no attempt to explore consumer definitions of health research and to align these with other perspectives. Consumer involvement has persistently been misrepresented as a method, when it can be more appropriately described as a *perspective* (comparable in some ways to a feminist perspective). Regarding consumer knowledge as expertise would require little translation, though it would require a shift in power and the forging of different models of health research that incorporate (or at least acknowledge) this perspective.

Forging different models of health research

To forge different models of health research that are capable of incorporating consumers requires that the research (and medical) community challenge the existing status quo that only researchers have a detailed understanding of the current knowledge base; are able to access other published knowledge; are trained in research methodology; can undertake the statistical analysis of data; and can write up the 'results' of research. Conceptually speaking, this epistemological challenge (Williams and Popay 1994) necessitates a reconsideration of what constitutes 'knowledge.' More practically, it requires that we revisit the construction of the infrastructure of health research, such as universities and the NHS, which contribute towards the continuation of expertise including accessibility to computer software and information technology (IT) facilities, existing research, other experts, and funding opportunities.

Drawing a parallel with the feminist perspective in research is illustrative here. As noted earlier, the dominance of positivism and empiricism forged specific representations, and partial accounts of knowledge that were then presented as generalizations (Haraway 1991; Harding 1991). Such accounts marginalized whole groups of people, notably women. For some feminists the social, political, cultural and economic domains, including language and meaning are saturated with male power (Spender 1980). As such, the work of women and their voices are hidden. To illuminate the work of women and thus, to explore wider social relations, feminist authors have published on the daily activities of women such as housework, reproduction and family relationships (Oakley 1974; Brown and Jordanova 1981; Griffiths 1988). Initially, the response to this new perspective was reluctance and hostility; combined with debate as to whether there could be feminist methods, as distinct from other methods used in the social sciences (Harding 1987). Central to the feminist perspective is the promotion of the voices of those who are disempowered, (in this case women, but this could also apply to the voices of patients) and to address the power imbalance in the relationship between those with power and those without (men and women; the researcher and the researched; patients and doctors). In this way, the feminist perspective challenges existing notions of research, especially positivist methods. It aims to address the power imbalance in the research setting/data collection, and to encourage reciprocity between researchers and the researched. Finally, it encourages reflection: rejecting the notion of objectivity and universal truths, and instead places value on the 'situated knowledge' of individuals (Haraway 1991), and to be aware that the scientific method encourages particular representations of the world.

Conclusion

Our motivation for writing this chapter is the belief that the conceptual and theoretical development of consumer involvement in health research is the only way in which this policy can be made not only palatable to the research and medical communities, but also possible in a practical sense. We have argued that consumer involvement might be facilitated by the construction of a transportable and standardized theory-method package that will bridge the gap that currently exists between consumers' and researchers' perceptions of health research (also illustrated in the case studies we present). Previous attempts to do so have stopped short of acknowledging some of the obstacles that we have highlighted in our analysis. However, the construction of such a package, or any attempt to move the debate forward, brings further difficulties, as we shall conclude this chapter by illustrating.

We have identified several key obstacles to consumer involvement, these are outlined below, with the questions the research community and consumers must seek to answer together in order to overcome them.

Health research and many of its researchers are steeped in a scientific method and infrastructure that requires a high degree of 'insider' knowledge

Given the dominance of the scientific method and the infrastructure within which research is conducted, it is unsurprising that it is difficult for consumers to penetrate the social world of research, and it is questionable whether this will ever be possible when researchers retain the responsibility for research and set the agenda (Cornwall and Jewkes 1995). Policy, literature and guidance repeatedly suggest that consumers can contribute to the identification of research problems and the formulation of research questions with little regard for this major obstacle (see Case Study 1). We suggest that in order to move the debate forward, there must be some attempt to clarify or investigate how and why the problems or questions identified by consumers might differ from those identified by researchers. In view of the power retained by the research community in relation to the conduct of health research, it is essential that we consider whether it is necessary for consumers to acquire 'insider' knowledge in order to attain a more equal relationship with researchers, and why this is so. We suggest that the processes by which consumers acquire such knowledge and the effects of any change in their approach to research should be carefully documented and examined for the insights they might provide into the merging of these two social worlds (see Case Study 2). This is particularly pertinent when considering knowledge produced by 'users' who are also academically qualified (e.g. Peter Beresford, Alison

Faulkner). How does knowledge produced by non-health service users, researchers, or consumer-researchers differ, if at all? And how is the validity of that knowledge affected by formal research training and acquired expertise? Finally, the impact of consumer involvement on the distribution of power and expertise in the doctor–patient and the researcher–researched relationships should also be addressed.

The term 'consumer' implies some form of agency and partnership
between researchers and consumers that at present is open to tokenism

A central tenet of our argument is that the research community must acknowledge the value of and integrate 'consumer knowledge'. However, as Peter Beresford (2000) has warned in the field of social work, integration in this way may only perpetuate the existing power imbalance:

> Even if they [social workers and theoreticians] were to address service users' perspectives, the issue would still be problematic. Many service users, including this writer, would argue that such theorizing cannot accurately reflect service user perspectives, because it remains part of a dominant discourse which has traditionally defined and continues to define service users in ways which they see as oppressive. If knowledge is not taken as given, then what we are actually seeing here are different and competing knowledge claims; those of social work theoreticians and those of social work service users and their organizations.
>
> (Beresford 2000: 497)

He suggests, 'social work theory building needs to take account of service users' own discussion about knowledge and their own theory building' (Beresford 2000: 497). He goes on to propose that theory building should include not only the knowledge of service users, but also the service users themselves, by giving them access to, and supporting them in theoretical discussion, and that postmodern approaches to multiple perspectives would facilitate this (Beresford 2000: 498–9). But Beresford's approach does not resolve the issue, as the question persists: *who* will define what qualifies as 'knowledge' or 'theory building' by service users? In the first instance, it is for the research community to consider what constitutes a consumer or researcher perspective, especially as making the distinction in the first place reflects the power structure within which research takes place. It would also be fruitful to analyse efforts to give consumers access to and support in their theoretical discussions, to see what form such access and discussions would take. Although this too would require the prior examination of what constitutes 'theoretical discussion' from the consumer or researcher perspective, since their conceptualization is likely to differ (see Case Study 1).

The type of knowledge that is common currency within health research
needs to accommodate the situated knowledge of consumers to forge a
consumer perspective

We suggest that it is helpful to view consumer involvement in a similar way to the feminist perspective: as a consumer perspective. This consumer perspective would place value on consumer input and views, and would encourage reflection on the impact that involving consumers has on research. Rather than treating consumer involvement as a new method, we urge researchers and clinicians to view it as a different way of seeing: to situate consumers' knowledge.

As with the advent of feminism, as well as raising questions about what constitutes valid research problems, the adoption of a radically different approach to consumer involvement that challenges existing power relations has significant consequences for *how* we define the problems, questions and techniques that we seek to investigate and to which we envisage that consumers will contribute. Consumer involvement challenges the perversity of the production of knowledge about health and illness, which has generally been produced in the absence of consumers' contributions, and saturated in biomedical frameworks. However, what this chapter hopes to convey is that it is not adequate to add consumers and stir (Harding 1987). For example, comments by a consumer on the language and the 'story' of a lay summary for a research project does not adequately reflect consumer involvement in a research project. If research and medical communities can acknowledge that it is not possible to separate the purpose of research from the origin of a research problem, then we can begin to unpick the components of research and begin to envisage the potential contribution of consumers. Consumer involvement in health research is required in order to develop and incorporate competing and different forms of knowledge; such knowledge cannot be considered to be knowledge or capable of incorporation without involvement; but, involvement cannot proceed unless different kinds of knowledge come to be considered knowledge.

As already noted, feminist work has contributed to reconceptualizing and challenging the existing dominant paradigms of scientific research and practice. Feminist inquiries into scientific research acknowledged that there is a body of activity called research (the method) and set out to redefine what research achieves (the production of knowledge) and how such knowledge is enrolled into different discourses. We suggest that consumer involvement can be viewed in the same way, as having the same goals, we would go further, and suggest that for consumer involvement to succeed, the research community may have to reconsider more fundamental questions such as: What is research? How do we do research? What other ways could research be done? And crucially, how can we redefine research in such a way that incorporates the involvement, perceptions and knowledges of consumers?

Throughout this chapter, we have argued that consumer involvement in health research requires more than policy guidelines that simply instruct researchers to 'involve' consumers. There must be an acknowledgement of the obstacles to involvement and wide ranging discussions of theoretical, and practical issues as they arise. And crucially, health research, in its widest meaning has to be able to move away from positivist leaning towards a more inclusive and tolerant framework.

Case Study 1: Mersey Primary Care Research and Development Consortium Workshop

The Mersey Primary Care Research and Development Consortium is funded by the NHS Budget 1, and consists of five primary care practices with the express aim of developing and facilitating a research culture. A workshop was held on the role of consumers in research as part of an open day to inform Consortium members about its work. A mixture of practitioners and consumers attended the workshop from the Consortium. The research experience of both the patients and some of the practitioners who attended was limited or non-existent. Workshop participants were invited to comment on what they thought health research was and to give suggestions for research that they thought should be conducted by the Consortium. Their responses alerted us to several issues that have consistently been overlooked or inadequately dealt with in the literature and guidance relating to consumer involvement in health research and are discussed below.

Conceptualizations of health research

It was apparent from the discussion in the workshop that for these consumer-participants, 'what is research' was blurred with 'research topics'. The patient-participants did not conceptualize research in terms of processes or methods, or even as a discrete activity, but in terms of topics and findings that they had heard about in different media. Thus, they made little distinction between issues relating to service provision, the provision of health/illness information and communication, and sharing of their experiences with other patients and carers. Such perceptions are at the very heart of our critique of consumer involvement in health research. As noted at the beginning of the chapter, the scientific method and its attendant techniques and models have developed over many centuries and are omnipresent within health research and represent specific ways of 'seeing'. It is taken for granted that the public/patients will be enrolled (or cajoled) into conceptualizing research in the same way as researchers, academics and practitioners. The scientific method will seep into consumer involvement, and by association scientific/health knowledge.

Research topics

The patient-participants raised a number of general and specific examples of service anomalies and failures, such as long waiting times for referral into specialist centres – to reconceptualize these as 'research topics' or 'research questions' from the discussion would be quite straightforward for researchers. In contrast, while the patients–participants discussed these as issues that required attention, they did not identify them as requiring 'research'. Thus, to derive research topics/questions from their comments would require the researchers to make a leap on their behalf, and this would surely introduce the researchers' priorities into the identification of research topics/questions. This is not a new problem for (qualitative) researchers, who are well practised in reflecting upon and documenting the ways in which they have influenced the direction and content of their research design and analysis. However, it raises the question whether it would be possible to formulate research questions without the influence of an experienced, and biased, researcher.

Consumer involvement in health research

The participants in the workshop indicated that they would want to be involved in health research. Nevertheless, when questioned about their specific involvement, they expressed ambiguity about how they could be involved. Such expressions are unsurprising. Nevertheless, if health researchers want to actively include consumers in a research project, then there has to be high degree of sharing of their 'insider' knowledge. For consumers to be truly involved in research then they have to be 'culturally drenched' (Featherstone 1991) in the language and discourses that are omnipresent within the health research community. Without such sharing, then there is an imbalance between the participants.

We suggest that any future involvement of the public in health research should take into consideration the impact of the researchers and consumers on the process of constructing topics and questions for investigation. Researchers must consider the impact of imposing their idea of what constitutes 'health research' onto consumers, and explore ways of integrating lay perceptions of health research into their methodologies, just as lay perceptions of health and illness must be acknowledged and considered.

Case Study 2: Steering group for the project 'return to work after mental health problems'

Consumers were involved in a study that looked at the factors that helped people with mental health problems to return to work. First, the researchers conducted a brief *consultation phase* prior to data collection. Second, the researchers worked *collaboratively* with consumers in the form of a project steering group. Third, towards the end of the project, participants and steering group members were invited to provide feedback on the analysis of the data and involved in its transformation into a script for a play written and performed by the production company AllTalk. It was hoped that this involvement throughout the project would lead to the use of language and concepts that were meaningful to potential participants and would be used in the research materials, such as information sheets and consent forms, and the script.

Nevertheless, there were limitations to this approach that we could not have anticipated. The information sheet and consent form were designed very carefully in a meeting with the steering group and a focus group during the consultation phase. It was agreed that the term 'mental health problem' was generally acceptable and would be used in descriptions about the project and in the information sheets and consent forms. We were using a wide definition of mental health problems to encapsulate not only medically diagnosed forms of 'mental illness' such as depression, but also 'lay' terms such as anxiety, stress and 'feeling down'. The recruitment strategy employed a variety of techniques, including snowballing. One unexpected consequence of this technique was that one individual who received the printed information about the study in the post rang the researcher (Krysia) and described feeling very upset that, according to the information sheet, he had been labelled as having a mental health problem. He did not consider his experiences to be 'mental health problems' and was distressed about others perceiving him in that way. The researcher took great care in explaining why the term had been used and tried to allay his fears about confidentiality. Despite his distress the participant was willing to be interviewed, though only on the condition that the consent form was altered so that it referred only to sickness absence and not to mental health problems.

We learned from this incident that, despite our best endeavours, not all problems can be anticipated, even when consumers are closely involved in the research process, and the development of the information sheet, consent form and interview schedule. On reflection, we consider that the individuals involved in the steering group, while providing a 'consumer perspective', were also comfortable with sharing their experiences and perceived themselves as someone with/who had mental health problems. In contrast, the participant we have described did not feel this way. This incident reveals the multiplicity of consumer experiences and perspectives, consumers' 'situated knowledge' and highlights how difficult it is to achieve consumer 'involvement' in any representative sense. Herein lies another problem: is consumer involvement supposed to be representative, and if not, what is it expected to achieve or contribute? Common criticisms of consumer involvement include its failure to be representative of 'consumers' or 'the public,' and the potential for the professionalization of consumers who are involved.

We suggest that researchers take care to define who they mean by consumer, and not to assume that this will be apparent – and to construct this definition as widely as possible to ensure that consumers along different points of the continuum are included. More importantly, researchers must consider what impact they believe involving consumers might have for their research, and to anticipate professionalization and desensitization.

References

Abercrombie, N. (1994) 'Authority and consumer society', in R. Keat, N. Whitely and N. Abercrombie (eds) *The Authority of the Consumer*, London: Routledge.

Baudrillard, J. (1988) *Selected Writings*, Cambridge: Polity.

Bauman, Z. (1987) *Legislators and Interpreters: On Modernity, Post-modernity and the Intellectuals*, Cambridge: Polity.

Bauman, Z. (1988) *Freedom*, Milton Keynes: Open University Press.

Becker, H.S. (1986) *Doing Things Together: Selected Papers*, Evanston, IL: Northwestern University Press.

Beresford, P. (2000) 'Service users' knowledge and social work theory: conflict or collaboration?', *British Journal of Social Work*, 30: 489–503.

Beveridge, W. (1942) *Social Insurance and Allied Services*, London: HMSO.

Bloor, D. (1976/1991) *Knowledge and Social Imagery*, 1st edn, London: Routledge and Kegan Paul; 2nd edn, Chicago: University of Chicago Press.

Bowker, G.C. and Star, S.L. (2000) *Sorting Things Out: Classification and its Consequences*, Cambridge, MA: MIT Press.

Brown, P. and Jordanova, L.J. (1981) 'Oppressive dichotomies: the nature/culture debate', in Cambridge Women's Studies Group (eds) *Women in Society*, Cambridge: Cambridge University Press.

Bury, M. (1997) *Health and Illness in a Changing Society*, London: Routledge.

Chalmers, A.F. (1999) *What is This Thing Called Science?*, Buckingham: Open University Press.

Clark, A.E. and Fujimura, J.H. (eds) (1992) *The Right Tools for the Job: At Work in Twentieth Century Life Science*, Princeton, NJ: Princeton University Press.

Clark, A. and Montini, T. (1993) 'The many faces of RU486: tales of situated knowledges and technological contestations', *Science, Technology and Human Values*, 18 (1): 42–78.

Collins, A., Kendall, G. and Michael, M. (1998) 'Resisting a diagnostic technique: the case of reflex anal dilation', *Sociology of Health and Illness*, 20 (1): 1–28.

Collins, H. and Pinch, T. (1993) *The Golem: What Everyone Should Know about Science*, Cambridge: Cambridge University Press.

Cornwall, A. and Jewkes, R. (1995) 'What is participatory research?', *Social Science and Medicine*, 41 (12): 1667–76.

Department of Health (1989) *Working for Patients*, London: HMSO.

Department of Health (1991) *The Patients' Charter*, London: HMSO.

Department of Health (1997) *The New NHS: Modern and Dependable*, London: The Stationery Office.

Department of Health (1999a) *Patient and Public Involvement in the New NHS*, London: DoH.

Department of Health (1999b) *National Service Framework for Mental Health*, London: DoH.

Department of Health (2000a) *Research and Development for a First Class Service*, London: DoH.

Department of Health (2000b) *National Service Framework for Coronary Heart Disease*, London: DoH.

Department of Health (2000c) *An Organisation with a Memory: Report of an Expert Group on Learning from Adverse Events in the NHS Chaired by the Chief Medical Officer*, London: HMSO.

Department of Health (2001a) *The Expert Patient: A New Approach to Chronic Disease Management for the 21st Century*, London: HMSO.

Department of Health (2001b) *National Service Framework for Older People*, London: DoH.

Department of Health (2001c) *The Report of the Public Inquiry into Children's Heart Surgery at the Bristol Royal Infirmary 1984–1995: Learning from Bristol*, Cm 5207(I), London: DoH.

Department of Health (2002) *Research Governance Framework for Health and Social Care*, London: HMSO.

Dixon-Woods, M. (2001) 'Writing wrongs? An analysis of published discourses about the use of patient information leaflets', *Social Science and Medicine*, 52: 1417–32.

Elston, M.A. (1994) 'The anti-vivisectionist movement and the science of medicine', in J. Gabe, D. Kelleher and G. Williams (eds) *Challenging Medicine*, London: Routledge.

Epstein, J. (1995) *Altered Conditions: Disease, Medicine and Storytelling*, New York: Routledge.

Ewen, S. (1976) *The Captain of Consciousness: Advertising and the Social Roots of Consumer Culture*, New York: McGraw-Hill.

Featherstone, M. (1983) 'Consumer culture: an introduction', *Theory, Culture and Society*, 1: 4–9.

Featherstone, M. (1991) 'The body in consumer culture', in M. Featherstone, M. Hepworth and B.S. Turner (eds) *The Body: Social Process and Cultural Theory*, Thousand Oaks, CA: Sage.

Fujimura, J.H. (1986) 'Bandwagons in science: doable problems and transportable packages as factors in the development of the molecular genetic bandwagon in cancer research', unpublished PhD thesis, University of California, Berkeley, CA.

Fujimura, J.H. (1988) 'The molecular biological bandwagon in cancer research: where social worlds meet', *Social Studies of Science*, 35: 261–83.

Giddens, A. (1998) *The Third Way: The Renewal of Social Democracy*, Cambridge: Polity.

Gilbert, N. and Mulkay, M. (1984) *Opening Pandora's Box: A Sociological Analysis of Scientists' Discourse*, Cambridge: Cambridge University Press.

Good, B.J. (1994) *Medicine, Rationality and Experience: An Anthropological Perspective*, Cambridge: Cambridge University Press.

Griffiths, M. (1988) 'Feminism, feelings and philosophy', in M. Griffiths and M. Whitford (eds) *Feminist Perspectives in Philosophy*, London: Macmillan.

Griffiths, R. (1983) *NHS Management Enquiry Report*, London: Department of Health and Social Security.

Grinyer, A. (1995) 'Risk, the real world and naïve sociology', in J. Gabe (ed.) *Medicine, Health and Risk: Sociological Approaches*, Sociology of Health and Illness Monograph 1, Oxford: Blackwell.

Hanley, B., Bradburn, J., Barnes, M., Evans, C., Goodare, H., Kelson, M., Kent, A., Oliver, S., Thomas, S. and Wallcraft, J. (2003) *Involving the Public in NHS, Public Health, and Social Care Research: Briefing Notes for Researchers*, 2nd edn, Eastleigh, Hampshire: INVOLVE.

Haraway, D. (1991) *Simians, Cyborgs, and Women: The Reinvention of Nature*, New York: Routledge.

Harding, S. (1987) 'Introduction: is there a feminist method?', in S. Harding (ed.) *Feminism and Methodology*, Milton Keynes: Open University Press.

Harding, S. (1991) *Whose Science? Whose Knowledge? Thinking from Women's Lives*, Buckingham: Open University Press.

Indyk, D. and Rier, D.A. (1993) 'Grassroots AIDS knowledge: implications for the boundaries of science and collective action', *Knowledge: Creation, Diffusion, Utilization*, 15: 3–43.

Irwin, A. and Wynne, B. (1996b), 'Introduction', in A. Irwin and B. Wynne (eds.) *Misunderstanding Science? The Public Reconstruction of Science and Technology*, Cambridge: Cambridge University Press.

Klein, R. (1983) *The Politics of the National Health Service*, London: Longman.

Klein, R. and Lewis, J. (1976) *The Politics of Consumer Representation*, London: Centre for Studies in Social Policy.

Knorr-Cetina, K. (1981) *Manufacture of Knowledge*, Oxford: Pergamon.

Latour, B. (1987) *Science in Action: How to Follow Scientists and Engineers through society*, Cambridge, MA: Harvard University Press.

Latour, B. and Woolgar, S. (1986) *Laboratory Life: The Construction of Scientific Facts*, Princeton, NJ: Princeton University Press.

Lave, J. and Wenger, E. (1991) *Situated Learning: Legitimate Peripheral Participation*, Cambridge: Cambridge University Press.

Lynch, M. (1998) 'The externalized retina: selection and mathematization in the visual documentation of objects in the life sciences', in M. Lynch and S. Woolgar (eds) *Representation in Scientific Practice*, Cambridge, MA: MIT Press.

McKendrick, N., Brewer, J. and Plumb, J.H. (1982) *The Birth of Consumer Society*, London: Europa.

May, T. (1996) *Situating Social Theory*, Buckingham: Open University Press.

Michael, M. (1996) *Constructing Identities*, Thousand Oaks, CA and London: Sage.

Miller, D. (1987) *Material Culture and Mass Consumption*, Oxford: Blackwell.

Mishra, R. (1984) *The Welfare State in Crisis*, Hemel Hempstead: Harvester Wheatsheaf.

Nettleton, S. (1997) 'Governing the risky self: how to become healthy, wealthy and wise', in A. Petersen and R. Bunton (eds) *Foucault, Health and Medicine*, London: Fontana.

Nicholls, S., Cullen, R., O'Neill, S. and Halligan, A. (2000) 'Clinical governance: its origins and its foundations', *Clinical Performance and Quality Health Care*, 8 (3): 172–8.

Oakley, A. (1974) *The Sociology of Housework*, Oxford: Martin Robertson.

Ogden, J. (1995) 'Psychosocial theory and the creation of the risky self', *Social Science and Medicine*, 40: 409–15.

Ong, B. (1996) 'The lay perspective in health technology assessment', *International Journal of Technology Assessment in Health Care*, 12 (3): 511–17.

Polanyi, M. (1973) *Personal Knowledge*, London: Routledge and Kegan Paul.

Royle, J., Steel, R., Hanley, B. and Bradburn, J. (2001) *Getting Involved in Research: A Guide for Consumers*, Winchester, Hampshire: Consumers in NHS Research Support Unit.

Schutz, A. (1944) 'The stranger: an essay in social psychology', *American Journal of Sociology*, 69: 499–507.

Spender, D. (1980) *Man-Made Language*, London: Routledge and Kegan Paul.

Strauss, A. (1978) 'A social world perspective', *Studies in Symbolic Interaction*, 1: 119–28.

Thorne, L., Purtell, R. and Baxter, L. (2001) *Knowing How: A Guide to Getting Involved in Research*, Exeter, Devon: Folk.Us, Exeter University.

Williams, G. and Popay, J. (1994) 'Lay knowledge and the privilege of experience', in J. Gabe, D. Kelleher and G. Williams (eds) *Challenging Medicine*, London: Routledge.

Williams, S.J. and Calnan, M. (1996) 'Modern medicine and the lay populace: theoretical perspectives and methodological issues', in S.J. Williams and M. Calnan (eds) *Modern Medicine: Lay Perspectives and Experiences*, London: UCL Press.

Wynne, B. (1991) 'Knowledge in context', *Science, Technology and Human Values*, 16: 111–21.

Wynne, B. (1996) 'Misunderstood misunderstandings: social identities and public uptake of science', in A. Irwin and B. Wynne (eds) *Misunderstanding Science?*, Cambridge: Cambridge University Press.

Chapter 6

Foster carers undertake research into birth family contact

Using the social action research approach

Jennie Fleming

Introduction

This chapter discusses social action research as a methodology that encourages those affected by or with an interest in the issues being researched (be they service users, community members, service providers, managers etc.) to identify issues for attention and have an active role right through a research project. It introduces the ideas behind social action research and shows how the approach was used in a research project with a group of foster carers.

What is social action research and where does it fit in with other models of research?

Kemshall and Littlechild (2000: 7) write that user participation has become a 'key issue in much current social work and social policy literature'. They suggest that research 'has the potential to objectify and stigmatise on the one hand, or to promote user participation and involvement on the other'. There are a range of degrees of involvement along a number of dimensions, from user controlled research (Beresford and Evans 1999; Fisher 2002; Evans and Fisher 1999) to non-participation where people are passive givers of information (most 'traditional' research). Beresford (2002: 96) identifies two different key ideological drivers for promoting service user involvement in research – 'consumerist' and 'democratic' approaches, which are based on different philosophical and ideological stances. He suggests that both have strengths and weaknesses. The democratic approach, however, has a commitment to personal and political empowerment and concern with bringing about direct change in people's lives through collective as well as individual action.

Service user or wider involvement is often linked with emancipatory or empowerment research, though it is not automatically so. Evans and Fisher (1999) recognize that service users need to be the ones who identify the need for the research, rather than joining in on research projects that are identified by academics. They write that a key question of the (emancipatory) model is how far the research can be emancipatory if it does not originate from the people affected and conducted under their control.

The Centre for Social Action (CSA) at De Montfort University, Leicester, has been involving service users and community members – those affected by the issues – in the research process for a long time. Early examples of this include a community consultation in the Somali community in Tower Hamlets (Gulaid et al. 1995) and the Black Community Safety Project (Saini 1997) both of which employed, trained and supported community members as researchers.

The social action research process starts with open-ended inquiry; social action researchers do not start with preconceived ideas and concepts, rather we work with all people with an interest in a issue or project to identify the focus of the research. These groups are involved in the refinement of the objectives for research, in the formation of methods and in the interpretation of the data collected. We look to establish a collaborative method with all people affected involved in the research process (see Fleming and Ward (1999) for a more detailed explanation of social action research).

There are three main points that identify social action research. First, as far as possible, the agenda is defined by those affected by or with an interest in the issue. Second, research is based on partnership between academic researchers and these groups. Finally, it is based on a recognition that all people have the capacity to be creative and be part of creating change. It is a collaborative method throughout.

It is the aim of social action research to negotiate with these groups to optimise their involvement in each situation. While there are many different degrees of involvement, there does seem to be a relationship between the extent of involvement in the research process and its capacity to serve an empowerment function. It is important that we listen to people about the level of involvement they feel is appropriate. For example, in a project in Russia, young people with HIV/AIDS did not want to be the researchers, as they did not wish to identify themselves in very prejudiced communities. They did, however, set the parameters of the research, decided on and developed appropriate methods and suggested how to make contact with people.

Social action research focuses on qualitative methods, as these allow for subtleties and differences of opinion to emerge. The data collected in social action research provide rich and vivid descriptions of people's lives and the clear insights that they alone can give into the difficulties and opportunities they experience.

Lloyd (1997) writes that for research to question the status quo is not enough. Oliver (1992) and Zarb (1992) believe the issue of real importance in research is 'whether research results in any material improvements'. Social action research is focused on change. Research is not an end in itself; the description of a problem, issue or situation is only the start, and research should provide an agenda for change.

Foster carers as service users?

Foster care is a vital activity in which children who cannot live at home for both short and lengthy periods are looked after in the homes of others. Foster care is the term used to cover the wide range of activities undertaken by those who care for other people's children, usually with the state acting as intermediary between the child's natural family and those given the responsibility for the care of its children (Ruegger and Rayfield 1999). Whether foster carers are service users or providers, or indeed both, is much debated. Clearly, foster carers are involved in the *provision* of services to children and families. Foster carers are now trained, receive a level of payment and, in some way, it is seen as a professional vocation and a challenging occupation (Ruegger and Rayfield 1999).

However, many people also talk of foster carers as being service users. Much research around foster care shows carers do not feel they are treated as partners by social workers. They are often excluded from decision making even when they have to carry out the decisions (Social Care Institute for Excellence (SCIE) 2003). There is much literature that discusses the lack of support for foster carers and very much views them as service users (Fisher et al. 2000; McDonald et al. 2003).

The group of foster carers in Birmingham that undertook the research in question did not accept the label of service user. They were aware that they were considered and called service users by the Social Services Department, and more widely, but it was not a label they owned. However, foster carers, and this research confirmed this, are in a relatively powerless position compared to service managers, social workers and the courts. They often find themselves having to implement decisions that they have had no involvement in making. The level of power people have in a situation is one of the key elements in a definition of service user in a SCIE publication (Levin 2004). The ambiguous role of foster carers and how one group relates to others in 'service user' and empowerment research is an issue in the example below.

The research project

The CSA was approached by Birmingham Foster Carers Association (BFCA) to help them with a research project they wanted to undertake. The two organizations had done work together before. The idea for the research project came from BFCA, who had been concerned about how birth parent contact was organized in the authority for some time. When safety was not an issue, foster carers were expected to receive birth parents into their homes for contact, and supervise it, regardless of the particular circumstances of the child and their birth relatives. The foster carer's home was assumed to be the place of contact. For many, this was a contentious issue, as they felt the specific issues in each case were not being adequately considered. BFCA was finding that carers were increasingly raising concerns about contact and its supervision. They recognized it was a complex issue, with many different perspectives involved. The committee decided to attempt to research the matter more widely.

The organization felt they would need some assistance to undertake the research. They believed that, as foster carers with the relevant knowledge and experience, they were well placed to be the researchers. However, they wanted the research to be credible with people in the authority, so that it could form the basis of change in how contact was organized. So, they approached the CSA to help them with the project.

Together, the two organizations developed a proposal for the research. BFCA submitted the application to the local lord mayor's charity committee, on his suggestion, and were granted money to undertake the research. The aim of the contract between CSA and BFCA can be summarized as: to train, support and supervise a research study to be undertaken about the organization of access visits by birth families to children in the foster home (from proposal document).

Once the money had been received, the committee asked its members for volunteers to be involved in the research. Initially, there were nine, which later dropped to seven and by the end of the project there were five people left. This dropout reflects the busy and stressful lives that many foster carers live. The seven researchers involved were four women and three men, of whom three were from black or ethnic minority groups. They were all very experienced foster carers and had experience of both short-term and long-term foster placements and had fostered children from birth to 16 years old (Manners et al. 2000).

The training

The CSA devised a training programme with the researchers. The training was experiential and participative. It was based on recognition of the wealth of experience in the group as the potential researchers were the experts in fostering and issues around contact. The CSA brought skills and experience too because we are experienced in participative and qualitative research. The training took the foster carers through a process that examined what they wanted to find out, who they needed to talk with to find it out and what methods might be best for them to find it out.

There were six training sessions. The first considered different approaches to research and what they wanted their research to be like. Some of the things they identified as being key to how they wanted their research to be were: interesting, beneficial, not too time consuming, valuing people's opinions, not to judge people, put people at ease, credible and to bring about good results. They also listed all the things they would like to find out, who they would need to contact and what research methods they might use. The next session considered the pros and cons of different methods of collecting information from different groups of people. They were keen to include the views of children, both those who were fostered and the children of the foster carers. Obviously, they were skilled and experienced in working with children but they still gave very careful consideration about how to best involve children and get their views. Much thought was also given to how birth parents might view foster carers asking them questions about contact visits. Role-play was used to raise and discuss a number of issues. These included the qualities needed by a researcher, what people needed to know before agreeing to take part and how to respond to situations that might occur in interviews (e.g. people starting to tell more of their personal circumstances than was perhaps appropriate or raising issues that needed to be complaints or involved child protection issues). The later sessions covered such topics as safety, how to introduce the research to people, getting consent to participate, recording as well as practical arrangements.

As the training was happening, simultaneously, the research was being constructed. In the sessions, decisions were made about who to include, what to ask them and guided conversation schedules were created and practised. Telephone approaches and interviews were role-played and, in the course of this, introductions were scripted, guidance on good practice and safety were drawn up and letters to people asking them to take part were written.

By the end of the training, the group of researchers had decided to interview foster carers, children who were being fostered, children of foster carers, birth parents and social workers. They chose to use individual interviews for all groups and, in addition, group interviews with some social workers. In keeping with the social action approach, they wanted to use an information collection method that allowed the people they were speaking with to talk about things that were important to them. They were well aware of the fact that, as foster carers, the issues of contact visits affected them but that the others they would be speaking to were affected as well, and that they would most probably have a different view point from them. The foster carers themselves wanted to recognize the people they were speaking with as experts in their own lives. They did not want to prescribe, beyond broad themes, what people could tell them. To this end, they devised a guided conversation schedule, with broad topics for discussion.

The steering group

Alongside the training and the decisions the researchers were making, a steering group was established. This included a committee member of BFCA who was not directly involved in the research, a representative from the researchers, the research adviser from the local authority Social Services Department and the researcher from CSA. Its remit was to guide and support the research work. Working closely with the researchers, decisions were made about, for example, the age range of children to be included, the size and make-up of the sample and methods for making contact with people. The worker from the local authority also took on the role of liasing and communicating with the Social Services Department, facilitating access to information.

The research

Once the training sessions were completed, the research adviser from the Centre continued to meet regularly with the researchers to offer advice and support and discuss and develop plans to overcome difficulties. The biggest problem that the research faced was getting in contact with people to ask if they would participate in the research. Contact with foster carers and their children was relatively easy. However, making contact with and getting permission to talk with fostered children and birth parents was a real challenge. The researchers and the steering group recognized that making contact with these groups was never going to be easy, and both groups of people put a lot of time, effort and creativity into thinking of suitable ways to do so. Initially, social workers were asked to identify birth parents who fitted the agreed criteria and to ask them if they were to willing to take part and give them a letter they could return to BFCA. In practice this did not work. A number of other routes were tried before it was agreed that foster carers who met birth parents on contact visits would ask them if they would consider taking part and give them the letter. This was an approach the researchers had originally rejected as they did not want the approach to be made via the foster carer because, despite giving reassurances, they were concerned parents would feel obliged to take part.

The difficulties experienced in getting in contact with people resulted in the research taking much longer than had been intended. Researchers spent a lot of time and effort in trying to get in contact with people. This had profound implications for their rate of pay. They had agreed to receive a fixed fee each for their work and, as the project took longer and longer, this meant the payment was much less generous than originally intended.

The foster carers were very concerned that their research should be of a high quality and that their closeness to the topic should not influence their work. They each tape-recorded and transcribed all their own interviews. After they had all done two or three interviews, they then swapped tapes and transcriptions with another researcher, who listened to the tape, made suggestions for how people could improve their interview technique and verified that the transcripts were accurate.

Analysis and report writing

It was agreed at the training sessions that one person would be responsible for writing the report and producing drafts for the group to comment on. This person received a slightly higher fee. However, everyone wanted to be involved in the analysis of the information collected. Once all the interviews were completed, all the researchers read the transcripts of all the interviews. The research adviser then facilitated a number of meetings where themes from the data were identified and commonalities and differences discussed. Everything was recorded on flipcharts and, ultimately, a plan for the report was developed from these discussions. The foster carer who wrote the report took the reams of charts away and drafted the report, which was then discussed and altered until everyone was happy that it reflected the breadth and depth of opinions and experiences.

What was found

Walmsley (2004: 57) writes that academics are more interested in the process of participative research than its findings. She suggests this is because the goal of including people in a meaningful way at times 'threatens to engulf the very real need for significant contents and outcomes'. The members of BFCA were emphatic that they wanted this research to be used to change things and improve the circumstances of birth parent contact, so the findings and their ability to influence decision makers were crucial. For this, process *was* important, but most definitely not at the expense of content. For this reason, a summary of the findings of the research follows.

Everybody reported some difficulty with the experience of birth parents and relatives coming to the foster home on visits. Foster carers having to sometimes supervise visits and undertake assessments (for which they were not trained) were an issue for all concerned. No one said the foster carers' homes should not be used for contact with birth relatives; they wanted each case to be fully considered and the right decision made for individual children and their relatives. Most importantly, no group of people, except social workers, felt they were involved in decisions about contact. Most people also felt they were unsupported, though there were some exceptions to this when individual social workers were felt to offer support. Both foster carers and birth parents reported having had trouble claiming expenses involved in contact. Birth parents were the least aware of their rights concerning contact (Manners et al. 2000).

People had a range of suggestions for improvement to the systems and arrangements for birth parent contact, and this led to BFCA making recommendations that would help make the experience of contact more positive for all those involved. These concerned the improvement of the practical and legislative context of contact, increased levels of support, training and participation, to encourage the development of specialist venues and personnel to manage contact (Manners et al. 2000).

What happened as a result of the research

The report went to senior managers in the department up to director level, to councillors and a senior family court judge. It also went to foster carers associations, nationally and internationally, and to various academics. It was reviewed in *Community Care* and the *Guardian* and by the National Foster Care Association.

There were meetings between BFCA and the Social Services Department to draw up and implement an action plan based on the research, and many actions were carried out. Joint training on contact was set up with foster carers as trainers. The department invested in its own research into good practice regarding contact and undertook a feasibility study for contact centres. The BFCA committee also met with a family court judge to discuss court practice in relation to decisions about contact. All of which resulted in changes to practice.

Issues arising from research

The researchers were foster carers, but they were collecting information not only from their peers but also from others involved. It would have been quite possible for them to mirror the mistakes and arrogance of academic researchers. So the approach and method they used in their research is particularly important. In this case, the foster carers chose to use social action research where the researcher asks questions, prompts and probes, in a relationship of equality, as far as possible. Respondents, whoever they are, are recognized as experts in their experiences; not as passive subjects but active participants who have the right to speak out and be heard. The foster carers choose their methods to reflect this approach. They developed techniques that were flexible and interactive. They were relatively unstructured techniques and there were no predetermined outcomes in mind. They used open-ended inquiry, open questions asking people how they felt about contact, what their experiences were, what they wanted from contact and what the best conditions for contact might be in their opinion.

Power and methodology

There are many powerful critiques of conventional research (see for example Oakley 1981; Oliver 1992; Holman 1987; Beresford 2002; Evans and Fisher 1999). They challenge the model of research where the researcher is seen as the expert and respondents solely as sources of data with no role or rights.

This project involved the process of sharing skills and experiences between an academic researcher and the researchers on the project. This sharing was not an end in itself, but a means of them undertaking a piece of participative social action research themselves (Truman and Paine 2001). The nature of participation raises a range of issues about the power relations between different stakeholders in the research process and how each is able to influence the way the research evidence is created and used. Within this research project, the way research evidence was created and used was in the control of the BFCA, but not the other key groups involved.

Taylor (1997) reworks Holman (1987) to suggest the following benchmarks for participative research: Who owns the research? Who defines the issues? Who decides how the topic should be researched? Who interprets the findings? What role do respondents play in data collection? And, finally, what purposes will the research be used for? The answer to all these questions in the example given here was most definitely the foster carers. However, it is not that simple because the research involved a wider range of people than just them. This raises a question about the relationship of power between the social action researcher and those they are asking to contribute to research. In this case, the researchers were all being paid, albeit poorly. But power in research goes way beyond who is being paid to participate. Power is affected by status, role, knowledge, culture and importantly people's assumptions and perceptions. Compared with birth parents, the researchers could be seen to be in a position of power. However, when they were interviewing social workers, there was a different power relationship, where the social worker could be seen to be in a more powerful position.

It is simplistic to view power as a fixed, binary concept (Humphries 1994). Foucault's (1980) theory of power suggests that power can never be absolute and is not a commodity that is possessed by people. Ward (1999) writes:

> Consideration of Lukes and Foucault enables us to move beyond 'zero sum' conceptions of power and empowerment – empowerment as something given and received from person to person, so that one person's empowerment must be another person's oppression.
>
> (Ward 1999: 51)

He goes on to say that 'empowerment must be allied to a commitment to challenging injustice and in particular oppression.' These are two important considerations in the research project undertaken by BFCA. They were committed to benefits for all involved via the improvement of contact visits and facilities (Humphries 1994).

The BFCA research used co-learning in their project; 'users and researchers emphasise their knowledge to create new understanding and work together to form action plans with researcher facilitation' (Shaw and Lishman 1999: 220). The research proposal was negotiated between BFCA, CSA and funders. The foster carers were involved from the outset, they had the idea and came to ask the centre to be involved. They formulated the problem, devised how to explore it and had ownership of findings. The foster carers' conceptualization of the problem came not only from their personal experiences but also from their knowledge and observation of the effects of contact in the foster home on the children fostered, their parents and their own children.

BFCA members were the researchers and so had to consider how to share power with their respondents. They did this by taking great care in how they constructed their research, their approach, methodology and methods. However, the reality is that others were still asked to join a process where the research issue and methods have largely been determined beforehand (Fisher 2002). In this project, there were a number of significant relationships where power could be exercised but, in each one, there was a commitment to address these issues and work in a way that was about the empowerment of those with the least levels of perceived power.

Evans and Fisher (1999: 102) suggest what counts as knowledge is key for people 'whose experiences may be defined by research *experts* in ways which are neither recognisable to users nor conducive to improvements in their lives'. The BFCA researchers were well aware of this and keen to construct their research project in a way that minimized this possibility.

Conclusion

Evans and Fisher (1999) are helpful in enabling an understanding of the issues raised by this piece of research. They write particularly about research on disability issues, but their work has a valuable contribution to make more widely to participative or emancipatory research. They quote Shakespeare (1996), who talks of the need to resist the notion there is a single 'right' way to do research, and says researchers must reserve the right to independent judgement. They go on to say, 'professionals must learn to place their skills in the hands of service users'. In other words, it is not enough to know how to research; what is required is the ability to 'assist service users to participate in the research enterprise in an empowering way' (Evans and Fisher 1999: 112).

Social action research is based on a recognition that those affected by the issues in situations to be considered have knowledge and experience that is as important as that of academics. The issue is how to combine these two sources of skill and knowledge by making our research skills and expertise available to others, so that they can make informed decisions about research for themselves. Evans and Fisher (1999: 114–15) suggest this requires a degree of professional humility. Our experience shows that, with mutual recognition of the importance and validity of different skills and knowledge, a willingness to work as colleagues, and a commitment to the sharing of skills at all levels and facilitation of a participative process, partnership research is indeed possible, and can make a positive contribution to improving the situation for people and the services they receive in the health and social care field.

Acknowledgements

As always the research and, hence, this chapter depended on a number of people and it is important to name at least some of them. The researchers who worked so hard and with such commitment were Jane Cook, Steve Holloway, Jugal Kishore and Barbara Willis. Particular acknowledgement and thanks go to Roberta Manners because, in addition to her role as a researcher, she helped me enormously by reading and commenting on drafts of this chapter.

References

Beresford, P. (2002) 'User involvement in research and evaluation: liberation or regulation?' *Social Policy and Society*, 1 (2): 95–105.
Beresford, P. and Evans, C. (1999) 'Research note: research and empowerment', *British Journal of Social Work*, 29: 671–7.
Evans, C. and Fisher, M. (1999) 'Collaborative evaluation with service users', in I. Shaw and J. Lishamn (eds) *Evaluation and Social Work Practice*, London: Sage.
Fisher, M. (2002) 'The role of service users in problem formulation and technical aspects of social research', *Social Work Education*, 21 (3): 305–12.

Fisher, T., Gibbs, I., Sinclair, I. and Wilson, K. (2000) 'Sharing care: the qualities sought of social workers by foster carers', *Child and Family Social Work*, 5 (3): 225–33.

Fleming, J. and Ward, D. (1999) 'Research as empowerment: social action approach', in W. Shera and L. Wells (eds) *Empowerment Practice in Social Work: Developing Richer Conceptual Foundations*, Toronto: Canadian Scholars' Press.

Foucault, M. (1980) *Power, Knowledge: Selected Interviews and Other Writings*, New York: Pantheon.

Guliad, A., Ismail, M. and Saeed, R. (1995) *Research into the Needs of the Somali Community in the City Challenge Area of Tower Hamlets*, Leicester: Centre for Social Action.

Holman, R. (1987) 'Research from the underside', *British Journal of Social Work*, 17: 669–83.

Humphries, B. (1994) 'Empowerment and social research: elements for an analytic framework', in B. Humphries and C. Truman (eds) *Rethinking Social Research*, Aldershot: Avebury.

Kemshall, H. and Littlechild, R. (2000) *User Involvement and Participation in Social Care*, London: Jessica Kingsley.

Levin, E. (2004) *Involving Service Users and Carers in Social Work Education*, London: Social care Institute for Excellence.

Lloyd, M. (1997) 'Partnership with service users: considerations for research', in R. Adams (ed.) *Crisis in the Human Services: National and International Issues*, Kingston upon Hull: University of Lincolnshire and Humberside.

McDonald, P., Burgess, C. and Smith, K. (2003) 'A support team for foster carers: the views and perceptions of service users', *British Journal of Social Work*, 33: 825–32.

Manners, R., Cook, J., Holloway, S., Kishore, J. and Willis, B. (2000) *Birmingham Foster Care Association's Research into Contact in Foster Homes*, Leicester: Centre for Social Action.

Oakley, A. (1981) 'Interviewing women: a contradiction in terms', in H. Roberts (ed.) *Doing Feminist Research*, London: Routledge and Kegan Paul.

Oliver, M. (1992) 'Changing the social relations of research production', *Disability Handicap and Society*, 7 (2): 101–14.

Ruegger, M. and Rayfield, L. (1999) 'The nature and the dilemmas of fostering in the nineties', in A. Wheal (ed.) *The RHP Companion to Foster Care*, Lyme Regis, Dorset: Russell House.

Saini, A. (1997) *'So What's the Point in Telling Anyone?' A Black Community Perspective on Crime in the Leicester City Challenge Area*, Leicester: Centre for Social Action.

Shakespeare, T. (1996) 'Rules of engagement: doing disability research', *Disability and Society*, 11 (1): 115–19.

Shaw, I. and Lishman, J. (1999) *Evaluation and Social Work Practice*, London: Sage.

Social Care Institute for Excellence (SCIE) (2003) *Fostering Success: An Exploration of the Research Literature in Foster Care*, Knowledge Review no. 5, London: SCIE.

Taylor, G. (1997) 'Ethical issues in practice: participatory social research and groups', *Groupwork*, 9 (2): 110–27.

Truman, C. and Paine, P. (2001) 'Involving users in evaluation: the social relations of user participation in health research', *Critical Public Health*, 11 (3): 215–29.

Walmsley, J. (2004) 'Involving users with learning difficulties in health improvement: lessons from inclusive learning disability research', *Nursing Inquiry*, 11 (1): 54–64.

Ward, D. (1999) 'Totem not token: groupwork as a vehicle for user participation', in H. Kemshall and R. Littlechild (eds) *User Involvement and Participation in Social Care*, London: Jessica Kingsley.

Zarb, G. (1992) 'On the road to Damascus: first steps towards changing the relations of disability research production', *Disability, Handicap and Society*, 7 (2): 125–38.

Chapter 7

From recruitment to dissemination

The experience of working together from service user and professional perspectives

Marion Clark, Helen Lester and Jon Glasby

Introduction

In this chapter, we will describe our experiences of working together on *Cases for Change*, a narrative review of adult mental health services, published by the National Institute for Mental Health in England (NIMHE) in January 2003. We will tell our story of working together in an essentially chronological order, and discuss the personal and professional costs and benefits of user involvement from both service user and 'professional academic' perspectives. These, as you will see, include not only the value of ensuring a user perspective throughout the work and the personal positive consequences of involvement for Marion, but also problems created by inflexible academic timeframes, lack of in-house support, academic practices such as the 'expert panel' system of reviewing work in progress and university employment regulations. We will conclude with a small number of practical recommendations, based on our experiences, to guide future researchers and service users who wish to work positively and productively together on a research study in an academic setting.

To set the scene, we'll first describe the research project that we worked on. Marion was involved, as the user researcher, in commenting on all aspects of the work, and leading on the user involvement chapter of the review. Helen and Jon were the 'professional academics' on the project. Helen has a primary care and mental health background and Jon has a social work/social policy background. Where appropriate, we will each give our own individual viewpoint, although most of this chapter has been written, as *Cases for Change* was, as a team effort.

Cases for Change

Cases for Change is a literature review and synthesis of the evidence on adult mental health services in England between January 1997 and February 2002. The National Institute for Mental Health (England) commissioned the review in winter 2001. The aims and objectives of the work were:

- to collate evidence from published and grey literature in both synthesized and non-synthesized formats on the evidence for reform in mental health services
- to review and synthesize all the information collected into key themes or issues
- to present the evidence in a manner that is accessible and useful to a wide audience including policy makers, service purchasers and providers, and users and carers

- to suggest cases for change drawn from this evidence base
- to disseminate the evidence in an effective manner
- to support and accelerate service improvements through spreading good practice, informing clinical governance and supporting the development of modern responsive health and social care services.

The timeframe for the study was short, although not unusually so for this type of work. We were awarded the work in December 2001 and the deadline for completion was August 2002. This meant that staff had to be appointed or seconded, the literature review completed, 658 papers and books obtained, classified, analysed and synthesized and the report (a series of ten booklets) written in seven months.

The relative speed of the work perhaps reflects the mental health policy context at that time. The National Institute for Mental Health in England was about to be launched (in June 2002). *Shifting the Balance of Power* (Department of Health 2001) had recently accelerated the timeframe for maturation from primary care groups to primary care trusts (PCTs) and *Shifting the Balance of Power: The Next Steps* (Department of Health 2002) gave these newly formed organizations, many of whom were trying to find their feet, specific responsibility for commissioning mental health services. There were also mental health targets to be met by PCTs in *The NHS Plan* (Department of Health 2000) and *The National Service Framework for Mental Health* (Department of Health 1999). One of the aims of *Cases for Change* was to help health and social care organizations negotiate their way through this policy maze and address local challenges armed with the evidence on what works and doesn't work in mental health. So, we needed to deliver a good quality review quickly and in an easily digestible format!

Our rationale for wanting active user involvement in *Cases for Change*

From the outset, we had proposed to employ a user researcher as part of the team and made this a central feature of our tender. This commitment was reinforced by Helen giving a joint presentation to the awards committee with a representative of a university-based 'users in research' group. There are, of course, a number of different and often interrelated benefits of involving mental health service users in research (and in teaching, service development and policy making). Our main rationale was:

- Users are experts about their own illness and need for care and will have viewpoints about issues grounded in lived experience. By definition, no one else, no matter how well trained or qualified, can possibly have had the same experience of the onset of mental illness, the same initial contact with services or the same journey through the mental health system. Users' viewpoints are therefore essential.
- Users may have different but equally important perspectives about their illness and care. Involving users in research work can therefore provide insights that prompt us to re-evaluate our work and challenge our traditional assumptions.
- User involvement may also lead to a new way of thinking about the nature of evidence itself, with what is sometimes seen as anecdotal experience given new validity through viewing it as 'human testimony'.

- User involvement may encourage greater social inclusion through providing employment and training opportunities (Sayce 1999).

In addition, we felt that having a service user as part of the core research team gave a strong signal about the importance of seeking different views. This was reinforced early on in the project as we quickly saw there was no one single 'case for change' in the literature – more a series of different stakeholders who have very different views. By including a service user perspective at the heart of the research team, we were able, as a social worker, GP and service user, to reflect some of those different voices and perspectives. We also decided that the initial title of the review, *The Case for Change in Mental Health*, should be amended to *Cases for Change* to reflect this.

As a result of the recruitment process, Marion was appointed to the post of user researcher at the end of the first month of the project. However, almost immediately things were not quite as straightforward as we had hoped.

An interesting start? The rhetoric reality gap in user involvement

Marion   I was really excited. After seven years of struggling with my mental health difficulties, I had finally got to the stage of applying for some work and actually getting it. But I didn't know what to do about the incapacity benefit I was on.

> 'Phone so-and-so [Employment Adviser],' said my friend. 'They'll know what to do'.

I got through to the person concerned and she took all my details. I told her I was going to do some research with academics based at the University of Birmingham. She asked what I had been diagnosed with, so I gave her my diagnosis, which included the word 'psychotic'. There was a silence at the other end.

> 'Ah,' she said, enunciating loudly and clearly, 'ARE YOU PHONING FROM UNIVERSITY HOSPITAL?'

I stared at the receiver and had to put it down as I burst out laughing. And this was the Disability Employment Adviser! Of course, it wasn't and isn't funny, but it gives some flavour of the kind of things that can happen to people who have or have had mental health difficulties when they try to get back into work.

Helen   From my perspective as the project lead, negotiating simultaneously with the university over appropriate payment and with the local Benefits Office over the implications for Marion's incapacity benefit was an enlightening experience and perhaps a microcosm of the frustrations that many people who are forced to rely on 'the system' experience. Poor internal communications and a lack of policy on employing someone who was perceived as 'incapable' by the state, but able to work as a paid academic, meant that I had the same conversation with a number of increasingly senior people in personnel and finance departments with no satisfactory conclusion.

Indeed, Marion had left the post before a solution was agreed and she was paid in the end in the same hand-to-mouth way that I pay students for occasional work in their holidays. This is not a good way to value a colleague. The Benefits Office was even more chaotic. I completed the same relatively long and complicated form by hand on two separate occasions, neither of which were apparently received or processed. I made four phone calls to try to clarify and speed up the process and sheltered behind my medical title when trying to persuade them that I was not incompetent and had indeed followed their rules. However, I was still made to feel as if the Benefit Office's lack of information was my fault, and I wonder how my psyche would have faired if my self-esteem had been low or I had rung up as Mrs, rather than Dr, Lester.

The work starts in earnest

Helen   By the end of the first month, the magnitude of the task was gradually beginning to dawn on us. It was perhaps even greater than we had imagined when we did the pilot search in preparation for submitting the project tender! The initial literature search found thousands of documents of which 658 were relevant to the project and were obtained. We used a classification schema to rate each article and were busy categorizing papers and books as they were downloaded or arrived from libraries and as inter-library loans. Jon's area of a small shared room was hidden under papers and box files and at times we all felt that the task was overwhelming. However, once we had organized and categorized the articles, the task felt more manageable and we began the time-consuming but interesting process of reading and synthesizing the literature.

We decided to divide the publications in the most pragmatic and useful way possible for commissioners and front-line staff. The ten booklets in the review were therefore focused on issues such as primary care mental health, inpatient care, community-based services, user involvement and partnership working, with clear signposting between booklets to make the links, for example, between user involvement and other aspects of health and social care.

Marion   For me, however, I felt I was doing too much too soon. I was very enthusiastic about participating in this piece of research, being fully convinced of the need for change and threw myself into it, heart and soul. But as I worked through the piles of literature (and there were 69 books and articles to read for the user involvement chapter in under four months), I began to lose sight of the wood for the trees. Since I felt I didn't know enough about the user/survivor movement, I also spent time researching that as well as reading the literature for the chapter. My stress levels began to mount. I was also working on my own in writing the user involvement chapter and didn't have anyone to discuss it with on a day-to-day basis. I felt responsible for everything. We had no fallback arrangements in case I became ill and could not continue. Eventually, I did, and I had to withdraw from the research. I suppose we could say that what was positive was that I recognized what was happening and was able to take steps to avoid any serious repercussions. However, there was not enough time to reorganize the work. The time allocated for the project meant that we were all quite pressurized into getting it done quickly. However, even becoming ill was a valuable learning experience for me. I was forced to sit back and reflect on what had gone wrong (i.e. that I had to stop work). The experience became part of my recovery as I realized I had been repeating the things that had partly at least made me ill in the first place. With this realization, I was able to take steps to make changes and go on to do other work in mental health.

Helen   As Marion describes, shortly before the end of the project, she became ill and was unable to continue working. We still had to complete the work within the tightly prescribed deadline, but finding personal capacity to take on an unexpected workload was difficult. Jon shouldered most of the additional work but as the project lead, there were anxieties related to missing deadlines and sadness that, as an individual, I had failed to provide sufficient support or indeed notice at a sufficiently early stage that Marion was finding the considerable workload difficult.

Jon   When Marion began to become unwell, I had two reactions: one personal and the other professional. On a personal level, I was sad that Marion felt under this pressure and concerned about what I individually and we as a research team may have done to contribute to this situation. In particular, it was hard to accept that a project that we had established with good intentions in mind had led to such a negative outcome for one of the team and a tough lesson that even well meaning attempts to involve service users may not always work. Professionally, I had already taken a lead on six of the ten reports and now had a seventh to write at very short notice. This increased the pressure on me substantially, and I began to fear for my own well-being as I struggled to accommodate this extra workload within very tight timescales.

Academic culture

Helen and Jon   The competitive culture of academia is an unforgiving one that is easy to assimilate as part of professional socialization and much harder to recognize as something that has significant limitations. It is possible that the focus on completing on time and in budget, and producing a review that would be of real value at the coalface, had in fact created pressures that 'professional academics' see as part of the role, but which are alien to someone returning to work and who needs nurturing rather than throwing in at the deep end.

A further example of academic culture, at least in terms of working on *Cases for Change*, was the function of the expert panel. The panel included acknowledged stakeholders in primary care, secondary care mental health, social care, and end users (including a PCT senior manager and service user). It met on two occasions (months three and five) to highlight documents published prior to 1997 that were key in developing the mental health agenda, advise on structure and synthesis strategies and provide specific written feedback on the final report.

The afternoon of each panel meeting consisted of a short presentation by the study team followed by discussion with the whole group on progress and future direction. At no time was the expert panel anything less than polite and encouraging of

Marion's role and ideas. However, some members voiced valid criticisms of, for example, the lack of an overall theoretical framework for the review, the number of exclusion criteria and the decision to report the findings using a largely structural rather than thematic approach. The suggestions were offered with academic certainty from senior and respected colleagues but could be perceived, particularly by someone with limited academic 'gladiatorial' experience, as undermining the project's value and the project team's worth.

Marion It is difficult for me to make an assessment of the expert panel, mostly because by the time I met the panel I was quite close to breakdown point. The experience could have been the straw that breaks the camel's back and I certainly did not find it a pleasant one. While recognizing the necessity of such an experienced group to comment on the integrity of a piece of work, I found it difficult to understand why, when dealing with mental health (of all subjects), the process had to be so stressful. I was surprised to find myself thinking that some of the comments of some panel members showed a lack of understanding of the realities of mental illness and also a lack of knowledge about the substantial contribution of the users' movement.

Benefits of service user involvement

Marion Whatever the difficulties outlined above in our assessment of user involvement in the project, the experience for me was overwhelmingly positive. Involvement in *Cases for Change* was a valuable and therapeutic experience on a personal level and provided a number of important opportunities for me, which were:

- the opportunity to interact with other people in the context of work
- the opportunity to resurrect skills that appeared to be lost from so many years of concentrating on recovery from mental breakdown
- the ability to acquire new skills and further knowledge
- the possibility of enhancing my self-esteem and self-confidence, both of which are severely damaged by the experience of having one's entire life called into question, which can happen when you fall victim to a mental illness
- the opportunity to earn some money
- the chance to apply the knowledge and experience gained from having been through and overcoming many of the difficulties caused by mental health problems
- the realization that other people are aware that lived experience is valuable and that your views are important: for anyone to recover from a severe mental illness is a triumph in itself, both for the person involved and for what he or she brings to the question, 'How did you do it?'

Although the above may seem like relatively short-term personal gains, in my view the significance of just a few people working together with the right attitudes is much broader. It's the familiar ripple effect of throwing a pebble into a pond.

Benefits from a 'professional academic' perspective

Helen and Jon   Working with Marion was certainly a valuable experience for us both on a number of different levels, not all of which were directly related to *Cases for Change*. Marion's significant contribution to the review ensured the process and end product didn't simply reflect our professional or academic agendas, but was grounded in the reality of someone who knew what it was like to try to negotiate 'The System'. Getting to know Marion and hearing her experiences was also thought provoking as health and social care professionals. We are part of the system that sometimes delivers poor quality care and, as such, cannot completely distance ourselves from her experiences.

In particular, we believe that who we are, our backgrounds and our training inevitably influence the way we see the world. When conducting a narrative review like *Cases for Change*, there is always a risk that we subconsciously pick themes and issues out of the literature that support our own preconceived ideas. By having a multidisciplinary research team (including a service user), we were able to guard against these dangers as much as possible. We could constantly test out emerging findings with the expert panel and with the research team as a whole, and were able to frequently check back to make sure that the claims we were making from the literature were a genuine reflection of what we had read. On several different occasions, the three of us each read the same article and took away a slightly different meaning, and it was important to be able to debate this in team meetings to help us develop and reflect a shared understanding of the key issues.

Lessons learned along the way

Helen and Jon   It is, of course, possible to look at how we organized the work and say 'You should have done this or that'. Well, no doubt we 'should' all be doing things absolutely correctly, but in reality we don't. There is always a gap between theory and practice; the exciting thing is getting involved in bridging that gap and finding ways of working in partnership that are beneficial to all the partners. However, with hindsight, there are definitely things we all agree we would now do differently. Lessons learnt along the way include the following:

- We should have discussed a more realistic timeframe with the funding body, particularly since we feel that one of the strengths of our bid that may have positively influenced our appointment was the stated intention of employing a user researcher.
- We should perhaps have been even more overt in the advertisement for the post about the nature and volume of the workload, and offered opportunities to attend relevant training run by the Staff Development Unit at the university before the post started, in, for example, speed reading or writing for publication.
- We should have held more regular team meetings (perhaps weekly rather than twice a month) since this would have allowed the team to 'gel' more quickly, to trust each other in expressing concerns about workload and perhaps to have

picked up the early warning signs that Marion was under pressure. It's interesting if not ironic that we were reading literature on the importance of partnership working, prevention and early warning signs but we were, at least at that time, unable to internalize the messages.

- We should perhaps have had a longer debriefing session and been more sensitive to the potential issues that the expert panel process raised.
- We should have negotiated contracts and salary scales with the university Personnel Department and investigated the impact of a regular wage on incapacity benefits before we appointed a user researcher. This is something that needs to be done thoroughly on at least one occasion within each institution and then regularly updated as legal requirements and employment law changes. It is certainly something that we have since explored as we've employed further user researchers in the Department of Primary Care mental health team.
- Perhaps most importantly, we should have appointed two service users to work together, rather than a single researcher. This would have enabled mutual support, both in terms of sharing workload and experiences, but might also have taken some of the pressure off Jon as he struggled to assimilate an extra day a week workload.

The issue of the behaviour of the expert panel is more difficult. From an academic perspective, the challenges posed by the panel, initially in terms of the structure and then the analytic framework of the review, were essentially helpful and illuminating. Although we didn't adopt all the suggestions, the process of defending our chosen approach helped clarify our thoughts and produce a more rigorous review. However, there are rules of engagement that might be usefully borrowed from other disciplines such as Pendleton and colleagues' (1984) rules, detailed below, which have been used as a guide to giving feedback since the mid-1980s in the primary care setting.

Pendleton's rules

- Clarify matters of fact.
- Person being assessed says what went well and how.
- Assesser identifies other things that went well and how.
- Person being assessed says what could be done differently and how.
- Assesser adds to this and concentrates on the 'how' aspects.
- Person being assessed describes how the feedback felt.
- All involved agree areas for further work.

Conclusion

Marion   For me, it was, overall, a good experience, and I very much enjoyed working with Helen and Jon. Having come from what was at times a rather lonely and isolated position, despite the best efforts of my husband, my family and friends and professionals, of struggling to get to the roots of my illness, it was wonderful for me to be working with other people whose interest was also to contribute to the work of improving mental health services and involving service users in that work.

Jon and Helen Working alongside Marion was a crucial part of *Cases for Change* and made the final report much more accessible, accurate and robust than it would otherwise have been without a user perspective. Despite all the problems, we are proud that we managed to work together as a team to produce such a major piece of work and hope that our different voices as social worker, GP and service user are reflected in the final document, promoting debate about the different perspectives that exist and the best ways forward.

Cases for Change was completed on time and was well received by the mental health community. We all attended the launch of the review at the NIMHE conference in Liverpool in January 2003 and watched with delight as the stacked copies of *Cases for Change* disappeared rapidly during the first day. Each of the eight National Institute of Mental Health regional development centres also distributed hundreds of copies and we had the great pleasure of receiving emails from colleagues who valued the pragmatic, down to earth and user focused approach we adopted.

We've also continued to work together since then. Marion and Helen, for example, are helping to develop meaningful user involvement in the Heart of England Mental Health Research Network Hub, Marion is reviewing a book for a journal that Jon edits and we are working together on this chapter and other projects. And that, perhaps, is the lasting testimony to our experiences of working together on *Cases for Change*.

References

Department of Health (1999) *The National Service Framework for Mental Health*, London: DoH.

Department of Health (2000) *The NHS Plan: A Plan for Investment, a Plan for Reform*, London: DoH.

Department of Health (2001) *Shifting the Balance of Power within the NHS: Securing Delivery*, London: DoH.

Department of Health (2002) *Shifting the Balance of Power within the NHS: The Next Steps*, London: DoH.

Glasby, J., Lester, H., Briscoe, J., Clark, M., Rose, S., England, E. (2003) 'Cases for change: a review of the foundations of mental health policy and practice', 1997–2002, Leeds: NIMHE.

Pendleton, D., Schofield, T., Tate, P. and Havelock, P. (1984) *The Consultation: An Approach to Learning and Teaching*, Oxford: Oxford University Press.

Sayce, L. (1999) *From Psychiatric Patient to Citizen: Overcoming Discrimination and Stigma*, Basingstoke: Palgrave.

Chapter 8

Consumer led research?

Parents as researchers: the child health surveillance project

Brenda Roche, Phillipa Savile, Daphine Aikens and Amy Scammell

Introduction

This chapter examines consumer involvement in a qualitative research study that focused on investigating parents' views of child health surveillance. We provide an overview of findings, a description of the consumer involvement and the experience of two of the parent-researchers involved, plus a discussion of the challenges and barriers that we experienced as a team in terms of consumer involvement. Finally, we try to provide an answer to whether this really was consumer led research. We hope that this will serve as a useful example to other research teams.

Background to the study

Programmes of child health surveillance are especially critical during the first year of a child's life and form the basis of ongoing health promotion programmes (Hall 1996). The nature of child health services has, in recent years, undergone significant change in terms of both design and delivery, moving away from provider directed models of child health surveillance towards a 'partnership approach'. Primary care child health services are striving to be more inclusive of parents in the process of monitoring and evaluating children's health (Hall 1996). Conventional wisdom suggests that such an ideological shift is both positive and welcomed. Despite this, the perspective of users of early child health services (parents) has remained largely unexamined. This study set out to do just this.

Overview of the study

This study examined parents' views of child health surveillance techniques and health promotion programmes offered in the first year of their child's life. The main objective of the study was to produce a description of child health surveillance from a parental perspective. In addition, we sought to identify the elements of current child health surveillance programmes that parents found to be beneficial, as well as those aspects that were considered unhelpful. Where services were seen as lacking, we sought to identify improvements or recommendations from our participants. Central to questions about the success or failure of any programme is the extent to which it accurately defines and targets the needs of a given population and this issue was crucial to our project.

We used qualitative methodology (focus groups and interviews) and our sample totalled 35 parents (34 mothers, 1 father). Participants were drawn from one of three general practice surgeries in Battersea, south-west London. The sampling was purposeful (Morse 1989) in that the study population were selected to provide a broad general knowledge of child health services from a variety of perspectives. The three practices' populations were characterized by differing levels of affluence and deprivation, ethnic and social composition and levels of identified health needs. Our starting point, or baseline population, from which we invited partici-pation included all participants registered with one of the three study practices who had a child under 1 year of age, or who were expecting a baby and were due to deliver and have at least one child health check within the time period of the study.

Parents were recruited using a variety of methods including postal questionnaire, contact through health professionals, approaching parents in local community organization and groups and snowballing techniques to ensure a broad sample reflecting the diversity of this inner-city area. Five focus groups and twelve individual interviews were conducted. All the data collected were tape-recorded and transcribed anonymously. The transcripts were analysed thematically.

Summary of findings

The findings of the research are mentioned here for interest. A number of main points were concluded. First, parents expressed more satisfaction at the eight week child health check, than the eight month child health check. They described the eight week check as being more comprehensive, medically informative and less bureaucratic. Critically, the eight week check appeared to provide parents with reassurance at a vulnerable point. Second, the desire and need for reassurance and support emerged as a key factor in what parents wanted and expected from health professionals in relation to child health services. Third, the health visitor emerged as a key individual in providing this reassurance and there was much support for the concept of a health visitor. Where parents described good relationships with a health visitor, it was clear that the health visitor had acted as a source of advice and provided support above and beyond her duty. However, most parents expressed dissatisfaction with their health visitor contacts, which they described as bureaucratic. Additionally, parents reported feeling excluded from accessing the services or support they perceived they required due to judgements made by the health visitor that were based on socio-economic markers such as quality of housing or income. Our study suggested that a lack of clarity over roles and expectations led parents to expect a different service than that which the health visitor provides and that crude socio-economic indicators do not provide an adequate means of assessing need and allocating resources. In such circumstances, partnership working between health professionals and consumers is rendered difficult if not impossible. The resolution of these issues should lead to improvements in parents' satisfaction with child health surveillance and child health promotion programmes.

The extra dimension . . .

While the description of the aims and methods is useful and the findings interesting and thought provoking, you are probably thinking that there is nothing remarkable about our study. However, we like to think that our study had a dimension that made it different from many others, a dimension that made it more robust and frank as well as more complicated and challenging. This is because our study had a strong degree of consumer involvement. Consumers informed every stage of the study, from design to dissemination, and the project itself would not have been possible at all without the involvement of three parent-researchers, who became part of the project team. This chapter discusses the stages of consumer involvement and issues (both positive and negative) that we faced over the life of the study.

Setting the scene: why consumer involvement?

There is an increasingly large amount of literature about the benefits of consumer involvement in health research and about the differing methodologies that various studies have successfully utilized. The increase in dissemination of this type of evidence is, without doubt, a good thing. This information will not be reviewed here, except to say that, in 2001, when this study was first conceived, evidence of consumer involvement was in much shorter supply and the idea itself was not fully recognized by the health research community as a useful, successful and/or necessary concept.

However, at a national level the views on the value of consumer involvement were more positive. INVOLVE (then called Consumers in NHS Research) had published a number of reports about the benefits of involving consumers in research and were able to provide advice to individuals interested in this area. The then NHS Executive London Region announced a call for research proposals under the Primary Care Studies programme. This programme was intended to fund research in and from primary care. Besides this, the main requirement was that projects display strong consumer involvement in their proposal and a commitment to including consumers in all aspects of the research process.

Stages of consumer involvement

In order to examine consumer involvement in the study, we provide a description of the different stages and the roles that the parent-researchers played in these. Difficulties and challenges are mentioned briefly but discussed fully in 'The big challenges and some barriers' section.

Project set up

The decision to involve local parents in the project was taken early on while the research idea was still being conceived and developed. The first parent-researcher to become involved was Philipa, who was approached by the lead investigator, her family GP. At first, it was not clear what shape her involvement would take. With little information on what consumer research meant, it was very much the beginning of a new adventure in health research experience for the growing team. Philipa soon found herself involved in the planning stages as the small team sought to prepare a research proposal that would be submitted to the funding panel – the Primary Care Studies Programme (PCSP) run by the then NHS London Region office. Several meetings followed, including a workshop for shortlisted studies, and finally after negotiation with the PCSP over capacity building costs and reassurance on academic support, the funds were awarded. Once the funding had been confirmed and before the project began, the lead GP and Philipa worked to 'recruit' a further five parents. The plan was to have two parents for each surgery that was involved in the research, making a total of six. This meant that each surgery would have a 'lead' parent and an additional parent that would assist him/her. However, finding these parents was not as easy as we had hoped. The recruitment came about in a fashion not unlike snowballing sampling. While the initial approach came from the GPs at each surgery, it was personal contact and reassurance from Philipa that secured the involvement of a further three mothers. It was felt that this was a sufficient number to proceed with the study.

As we began our study, our knowledge of consumer involvement was still rather basic but we were committed to making the study work. Despite initial apprehensions, and little understanding of the differences between qualitative and quantitative research, Philipa described why she felt it was so important for the project:

> Why did consumers need to be involved? Quite simply we know the service and have experience of using it. In fact we brought to the project considerable experience of using child health surveillance, the three lead parents had ten children between them ranging from 6 months to 14 years old.

Meetings

From the outset, the parent-researchers were included in all project meetings. These ranged from one-to-one sessions with the study researcher to full steering group meetings that included the academic partners, experts and primary care professionals from the three participating surgeries. They were interesting and useful but they were time consuming. Scheduling proved very difficult, with the study researcher often juggling competing demands of parent-researchers, academic partners, primary care professionals and venue availability.

The study team strived to make sure that the larger meetings that involved the wider steering group were accessible to the parent-researchers. This meant that they were held at the study team offices in Battersea and at times between school runs. Formality was kept to a minimum to encourage all to be able to input their views. However, there were times when clinical or academic points felt inaccessible and incomprehensible to the parent-researchers and this led on occasion to somewhat one-sided meetings. The study team attempted to counter this through the study researcher developing a close working relationship with the parent-researchers. They would often meet informally to discuss any problems or concerns. The parent-researchers were also invited to wider PSCP meetings in central London or to training events commissioned by the PSCP. While the ideology behind these was welcomed, the practicalities were lacking and it proved impossible for parent-researchers to engage with these events.

Training

The parents involved in the study would be key individuals in terms of data collection and it was planned that they would facilitate the climinate focus groups, the main method of collecting data. Focus groups were chosen because it was felt that they would produce more interesting stories and comments on child health surveillance, and the supportive atmosphere would encourage parents to share their views. Through having focus groups facilitated by parents themselves, we hoped to obtain a more accurate and truthful picture of parents' views of child health surveillance. We hoped that the parent-researchers would act as 'insider researchers' and provide a non-judgemental 'leadership' for the focus groups. We hoped that the data produced would be more robust and more reflective of what participants' experiences have been.

To enable the parent-researchers to facilitate and lead the focus groups, we decided that they would need training, which was arranged with the academic members of the study team at King's College London. The plan was to provide a background understanding in qualitative methods, discussion of focus groups and issues related to undertaking these and an opportunity to practice facilitating and to review this via video and make improvements to techniques.

At the outset, there were nine sessions planned and our academic team members suggested that the training could be accredited to provide the parent-researchers with a nationally recognized qualification such as a national vocational qualification (NVQ). However, difficulties in scheduling (a challenge throughout the study) meant that, in the end, the sessions were compressed into six, focusing in on key topics such as the risks and responsibilities that are part of focus group facilitation. Accreditation was discussed by the parent-researchers and decided against because it was seen as less important than being able to commit appropriate time to the study and the ability to undertake focus groups well.

Much of the training capitalized on what the parent-researchers described as 'common sense'. They described the training as encouraging them to draw upon their initiative, intuition and personality, which enabled them to feel comfortable with the idea of leading a group discussion. The use of role-play, which at first seemed a little daunting, helped them to feel more like researchers and gave them confidence to participate more effectively in the study team.

Data collection

The actual focus groups themselves were scheduled by the study researcher (Brenda) in liaison with the parent-researchers, two of whom facilitated each group. The study researcher also attended the groups to provide support and advice, if needed, for the parent-researchers. The parent-researchers described enjoying the focus groups immensely, and what felt like an awe-inspiring mountain to climb initially was quickly forgotten. They greatly enjoyed meeting people and networking, which was when their natural people skills came into their own.

Facilitating the focus groups inevitably involved frustrations and challenges for the parent-researchers, not least when participants did not turn up at the last minute and all those phone calls and attempts to schedule times were wasted. The dynamics of the groups were also variable. Some were comfortable and easy going, others more complex with individuals with strong voices who would have dominated the conversation if allowed. Keeping the tone reassuring, supportive and non-judgemental, and ensuring that different views were heard, were challenging. There were, of course, difficulties in finding venues where appropriate child-care could be provided, and some groups were held at the home of one of the parent-researchers. This provided a warm and welcoming atmosphere but could have proven an insurance nightmare. Again, a lesson to learn! Despite the difficulties, there were many amusing incidents. One tape clearly records the interruption of a parent-researcher's mother, who was staying in the house and wanted to chat, and another is drowned out for a minute by the use of a vacuum cleaner in another room.

Following each focus group, we aimed to debrief the data collection team (parent-researchers and study researcher). We talked about the group and any issues that had arisen. However, we did not have time to discuss comprehensively the dynamics that operated in the groups and how each of us functioned as facilitators. Additionally, it proved difficult to revisit this after transcription of the focus group tapes because this took considerably longer than anticipated. Full transcriptions were completed long after the actual groups had taken place. This was not ideal but reflects the issues of underestimating the capacity needed.

Data analysis

Data were analysed thematically once transcription was complete. The parent-researchers were not provided with formal training in this but were assisted by the study researcher, who showed them how to read and understand the transcripts and think about themes they felt arose from the data. All the study team members engaged in this process of identifying themes and, at a small meeting, everyone shared the themes they felt were most important. The top four or five issues and themes were agreed on and then the study researcher reviewed the data more formally and classified parts of the transcripts according to the different themes. This was undertaken using Atlas.ti, a software package that assists qualitative analysis. After this was complete, the whole study team reviewed the transcripts again and comments were made. The parent-researchers were able to engage in the analysis and some aspects of qualitative research appear to have been simplified through this.

Dissemination

All the study team members engaged in undertaking presentations of the findings at seminars and conferences. The parent-researchers were directly involved in several of these, commenting on the content of the presentations and actually presenting the work on different occasions. This provided an opportunity to improve presentation skills and learn more about computer software packages, such as PowerPoint. The difficulties related to presenting were again due to scheduling and timing. Often meetings involved a long journey and meant that arrangements had to be made to deliver and collect children from school and for after-school child-care.

Writing up presented a big challenge to the study team, not least because there were so many individuals involved in the project. Relatively early on in the study, we met to decide what route we would take with our publications and other dissemination activities. It was decided that the study researcher would lead on producing a general paper about the study, including the findings, and that other papers would subsequently be developed by other team members. We hoped this would ensure that the findings would be disseminated to a variety of audiences for maximum impact. The process of writing papers was complicated. It involved email circulation, imposition of deadlines, meetings, editing, more circulation. In reality, it was quite difficult to engage with and we would have benefited from more time to review articles and smaller numbers of individuals writing each paper.

Implementation

This study has now finished and the next stage is to try to encourage or facilitate implementation of findings. This is a complex issue involving time, capacity and liaison with groups of health professionals and service commissioners outside the study team. We are keen that parent-researchers are involved in this aspect of the project and are currently looking for ways to facilitate this and engage with the local health care community about our work.

The big challenges and some barriers

Expectations within the study team and group dynamics

Two of the most important issues we would advise any other team to address as early as possible are, first, expectations and assumptions about the roles of the different project members and, second, the group/team dynamics. Our parent-researchers were recruited informally and the study team aimed to provide support to them on a day-to-day basis, ranging from help arranging child-care and focus groups to answering questions about research methods and plans for analysis.

However, we did not develop job descriptions for the parent-researchers. Workload was estimated to be three to four hours a week for each parent-researcher for the duration of the study (fifteen months) but it was expected that this would fluctuate. We wanted to see how the consumer roles would develop over the course of the study and, in some ways, felt that additional formality, such as remits, job descriptions and stipulations about required knowledge and so on, would confine the parent-researchers to predefined roles. Philipa described very early on, at the proposal stage, how liberating it was not to be defined by a role but to wear a badge with just your name on it (not your job or place of work) when attending a meeting hosted by the NHS Executive London Region for all projects shortlisted for the PCSP awards. We liked the idea of the parent-researchers being able to contribute to the project at many different levels and not being defined as a 'consumer' but as part of the study team. We felt that being a consumer on a research study should offer the opportunity to move among all team members and across all areas of the project.

This worked to a certain extent. However, there were occasions when the role of the parent-researchers was less clear; in contributing to meetings on analysis and dissemination for example. In retrospect, simple job descriptions or remits would probably have been helpful. The key here, we feel, is to develop these sensitively with an emphasis on opportunities and choices, as opposed to requirements and skills. If this can be achieved, the remit and/or job description should provide consumers with confidence to fulfil their involvement effectively and enjoyably. Consumer involvement should be a negotiation and develop individuals' skills, not be a fixed role defined by an established academic project team.

Besides supporting consumers involved in research and clarifying their expectations, it is fundamental to address the expectations of other research team members. It is necessary to ensure that each team member understands that the contribution from consumers is valuable and important, and to disable the development of hierarchies of knowledge, where medical expertise or academic knowledge appears to invalidate the consumer perspective. This is, no doubt, no easy task. The key from our experience appears to be tolerance and focus on clear communication.

Communication

Communication or 'miscommunication' was an issue in our study and we would assume that it could have a major impact on all consumer research projects. Despite efforts to ensure 'consumer' friendly meetings, either at the PCSP or within our own study team, the reality could be quite different. The parent-researchers found themselves juggling with unfamiliar jargon and shorthand expressions commonly used in health research, from PCTs to NSFs (National Service Frameworks). At times, this was a source of great frustration. However, over time, the parent-researchers realized that although this was common, it was unintentional. It also became clear that the use of specialized terms were not exclusive to the research team. For example, while conducting focus groups, we identified terms and expressions commonplace within the world of parenting, such as 'The Red Book'. While this is familiar to those people with children, those without, such as two members of the study team, found the concept wholly unfamiliar.

The difficulties we all faced over communication taught us the necessity of open communication and brought to all of our attention the ways in which we all rely on specialized knowledge in different areas. Once we had recognized this, we focused on it as a source of strength as a team, rather than allowing it to become a source of anxiety. This allowed us to increase in confidence and progress onwards.

Payment/remuneration

Our study team felt strongly that consumers should be remunerated for their contribution to the study, as were all other members of the study team. Funding for this was costed into the research proposal but we had no clear idea of how much was an acceptable 'salary'. In the end, we made the salary comparable with a researcher salary pro rata. A clear job description here would probably have been helpful!

Support from the PCSP

One of the biggest challenges, surprisingly, came from the need to engage in the PCSP agenda alongside undertaking the research study. While the PCSP was committed to consumer involvement, organizational change within the Department of Health and delays in programme support and training meant that our project felt disengaged from the wider programme. Of the eleven commissioned projects, most were at least eighteen months in duration. At fifteen months, we were in a minority and felt under considerable time pressure to move our study forward.

As soon as our funding was secured, we were ready to access training and support for our parent-researchers (in research methods, the research process etc.) and for our wider study team (in consumer involvement etc.). However, there was considerable confusion over the commissioning of training and support, with the two teams charged with this remit unclear of their roles and project needs. When training and support did become available, we had already begun to provide and access our own. The training events that were held were generic and designed to appeal to consumers across all eleven projects. Letters sent out had pictorial representation and large clear font, which was beneficial to the study involving consumers with learning disabilities but to other consumers appeared patronizing and insensitive. This was, we felt, unrealistic and inappropriate. Consumers are not a homogeneous group and their needs are individual and project specific. Training events became impractical and more time-consuming than beneficial. We feel that this led to considerable dissatisfaction in many circumstances.

In addition to attending training events, the eleven projects were required to attend project programme progress meetings at stipulated points. The aim of these was to share experiences among the projects and facilitate learning around consumer involvement. This was something that the projects were keen to be involved in and it was welcomed. However, details of the practical arrangements were not thought through fully. Meetings were large and located across London. It proved impossible for our parent-researchers to combine these with the everyday necessities of school runs, work and so on. Additionally, many of the primary care professionals involved found it difficult to attend due to the need to reschedule clinics. Thus, while we tried to make sure that our study was always represented, individuals who stood to gain most from these shared events were unable to attend. This was compounded part way through the PCSP first year when reorganization at the Department of Health meant the demise of the regional offices and regional funding. This in turn meant that the PCSP, which was due to make a second annual call for proposals, and to provide support to projects over their entire lifetime (up to three years), also came to an end. Projects could no longer be supported by NHS Executive staff, the newsletter stopped as quickly as it had begun, and contact between the projects ended. We were left feeling detached and somewhat adrift in relation to the larger programme.

Timescales, scheduling and practical support

One of the most problematic issues for our project related to scheduling meetings and keeping within our timescale. Everyone on the study team and the wider steering group brought different areas of expertise and, therefore, had differing commitments and workload, from working on other projects to teaching to seeing and treating patients to looking after children and their families. We all needed to accommodate hectic lives, and the way we did this was by accepting that not everyone could or would attend every meeting. It simply was not possible. The study researcher spent a good deal of time liaising with the different team members and ensured that people were updated and could input even if they couldn't attend a specific meeting. This involved a lot of patience.

There were, of course, other issues to consider when scheduling meetings. All parent-researchers had the occasional need for child-care and there were issues involved in setting this up. Sometimes the study team would simply pay the child-care expenses but sometimes we had to employ a child-minder and find a child friendly venue where the meeting could take place with the children cared for on site. This wasn't easy and increased time pressures on the study. Additionally, we needed to schedule meetings at particular times that did not clash with school runs and this did not always fit in with other people's needs. With this juggling and scheduling taking precedence, our progress on the study inevitably slipped against our plan. Luckily, we were able to extend our study researcher's contract from other funds and press on to the end. However, this was a source of considerable stress for the team and illustrates the need for overestimation of timescales due to practical issues.

Food for thought

In conclusion, we would like to say that being involved in a consumer led research study was tremendous fun and a great experience. As we have described, there were challenges and difficulties that we had to overcome, some related to our own study, some to external factors and not all to do with consumer involvement. We feel that consumer involvement is a necessary component of research projects if we are to address appropriate research questions and interpret individuals' views correctly. To effectively involve consumers in research we feel there is a need to work through a few basic steps:

1   Involve consumers at an early stage and work with them to structure a role or remit for their involvement. Try to work out what consumer involvement might mean for your study and remember that consumers are not a homogenous group.
2   Discuss any concerns or queries with a group such as INVOLVE or Folk.Us. They have significant expertise in consumer involvement in research and are happy to advise or provide support.
3   Discuss remuneration and any expectations of time commitments. Remember to budget for consumers' remuneration within your funding proposal and base this on sensible estimates such as researcher's salary pro rata. Also, consider the impact that payment may have on individuals' other income, such as job seeker's allowance or incapacity benefit.
4   Introduce all study team members to each other early on and get an idea of people's other commitments.
5   Try to schedule meetings that are inclusive of everyone, varying meeting venues and times as necessary. However, also accept that ultimately, even if you are flexible, no times will suit all if you have a large team. Be prepared to hold sub-meetings and contact people to let them know outcomes of meetings, or to ask for items for inclusion, if they are unable to attend. Assume that this will be at least twice as time-consuming as you think it should be!

6   Ascertain and set up any support or training that consumer team members will need well in advance. It may be appropriate for them to join generic research training but it may be that very specific training or support is needed and this will be more difficult to arrange and more expensive to provide. If the funder or sponsor of the study provides training and support, ensure that this is accessible, timely and appropriate. Make sure you have a contingency plan should this not work out.

7   Try to include consumers at each stage and budget to provide opportunities to attend conferences or meetings where possible. This means that their involvement will be more meaningful and will provide skills beyond the research process. For example, if we had not attended the INVOLVE conference in Harrogate, this chapter would not have been proposed or written.

8   Evaluate your consumer involvement and try to get feedback from the consumers on how things work. Ensure that you have the capacity and time to respond to these and make the necessary changes.

Conclusion: consumer led research?

So, in summary, was this study a consumer led research project? We feel that the answer to this somewhat depends on the interpretation of 'consumer led research'. We would say that consumer involvement was integral to the progress and success of the study and we do view this study as a success in that it elicited a variety of views from local Battersea parents on child health surveillance. This project was not totally designed and undertaken by consumers but the parent-researchers were involved at each stage of the process and were part of the study team. They led the data collection and won the confidence of the participants in a way that health professionals or external researchers may not have been able to. In this respect, we feel that the data produced from the study are more robust and valid. We feel that without the parent-researchers, this study would have been very different and in this respect they have led the project in many areas. The key issue for us as a team is that it is an example of collaboration and overcoming difficulties.

There will be different approaches to consumer involvement suitable for different projects and different populations but involvement at an early stage and a recognition of consumers expertise in a project area will mean that more consumer led research is possible. We are very pleased to have been able to undertake this study and hope that we will be able to build on and learn from our experiences of consumer involvement. We would recommend that all research teams endeavour to conduct consumer led research or increase consumer involvement in their projects. It is amazing what we can all learn from the process.

Acknowledgements

We would like to thank many people for their support during the course of the study. First, all our participants for their time and their views. Second, the other members of our project team, Susan Fitzpatrick, our third parent-researcher, and Adwoa Bolliston, our fourth parent-researcher, who had to leave the study early, Niki Salt, the lead investigator, Mary Malone and Sarah Cowley, our academic partners from King's College London. Third, the members of our steering group, in particular David Elliman, Helen Bedford, Rosie Savage and Jenni Ellingham. And finally, all the staff at the three practices who assisted in the project. The study would not have been possible without teamwork.

References

Hall, D.M.B. (ed.) (1996) *Health for All Children*, 3rd edn, Oxford: Oxford University Press.
Morse, J.M. (1989) *Qualitative Nursing Research: A Contemporary Dialogue*, London: Sage.

Further reading

Baxter, L., Thorne, L. and Mitchell, A. (2001) *Small Voices, Big Noises: Lay Involvement in Health Research – Lessons from Other Fields*, Folk.Us, Consumers in NHS Research, Exeter: Washington Singer Press.
Buckland, S. and Entwistle, J. (2000) *Suggested Guidance for Grant Applicants for Involving the Public in Research*, Eastleigh, Hampshire: INVOLVE (updated March 2004).
Nilsen, E.S., Myrhang, H.T., Johansen, M., Oliver, S. and Oxman, A.D. (2004) *Interventions for Promoting Consumer Involvement in Developing Healthcare Policy and Research, Clinical Practice Guidelines and Patient Information Material* (Protocol for a Cochrane Review), in The Cochrane Library, issue 3, Chichester: John Wiley.
Oliver, S., Clarke-Jones, L., Rees, R., Milne, R., Buchanan, P. and Gabbay, J. (2004) 'Involving consumers in research and development agenda setting for the NHS: developing an evidence-based approach', *Health Technology Assessment*, 8 (15), Southampton: National Coordinating Centre for Health Technology Assessment (NCCHTA).

Chapter 9

Consumer involvement in cancer research in the United Kingdom

The benefits and challenges

Tony Stevens and David Wilde

with contributions from David Kirby, Derek Stewart, Dawn Wragg, Sam Ahmedzai, David Cunningham and Janet Darbyshire

Introduction

Cancer is a major, and increasing, disease burden that affects one in three of the United Kingdom population who will at some point be diagnosed with the disease. It accounts for 26 per cent of all male and 22 per cent of all female deaths, with survival rates significantly lower than most European countries. It is among the three leading causes of death at all ages except for pre-school children (Wanless 2002). Total UK research spend on cancer is estimated at between £450 million and £500 million per annum (National Cancer Research Institute (NCRI) 2002). Following several policy initiatives, a number of national organizations have been created since the late 1990s to co-ordinate and integrate cancer research within the United Kingdom. Part of their remit is the involvement of consumers. We aim to contextualize these initiatives, to outline the current opportunities for consumers and to identify the key challenges that remain.

The changing environment of health care and its impact on research

In the United Kingdom nowadays, there is an increasing trend towards a more democratic provision of health services, with a strong emphasis placed upon citizenship predicated upon individual rights, community responsibility and social justice. As citizens and taxpayers, consumers are increasingly asserting their rights to have their voices heard in relation to how budgets are allocated and how research priorities are identified. Furthermore, the growth and influence of consumer groups, with agendas focused increasingly upon empowerment, has begun to change the way that patients perceive themselves – less as compliant recipients of health care but as individuals capable of making their own judgements about their choices for care and treatment. There is also evidence to suggest that the ways patients are communicating with the medical profession are changing and the passive patient/active doctor is becoming less common (Guadagnoli and Ward 1998). Some commentators have argued that these developments are essentially about the politicization of health care and challenging decision making monopolies (Entwistle et al. 1998).

The model of health conceptualized by the World Health Organization offers two distinct paradigms – disease, which is defined in terms of 'a physiologic and clinical abnormality', and illness, defined as the 'subjective experience of the individual' (Ong

1996). It has been argued that developing a consumer perspective expands this objective versus subjective (disease versus illness) taxonomy with a more holistic interpretation of health (Entwistle et al. 1998). By bringing the expert in terms of their own illness (the consumer) into contact with the experts in terms of the clinical interpretation of the disease (the health care professionals), the opportunity exists to exchange ideas and develop new insights. Consumers become more informed about the processes of disease and the professionals gain deeper insight into the experience of being ill.

The evolving trend towards a more collaborative approach, with redefined roles reflecting implicit challenges to professional knowledge, is affecting the ways that health professionals are conceptualizing and conducting research. The view that professional experts are the best judges of where research activity should be focused is being tempered by the rationale that 'patients should decide which research is conducted, help to plan the research and interpret the data and hear about the results before anyone else' (Goodare and Smith 1995: 1277). Within research, these developments present greater scope for prioritizing studies investigating issues that are important for consumers, for ensuring study designs incorporate outcome measures that have salience for consumers, for establishing procedures to feedback and disseminate results to consumers, and helping with the application of research findings into clinical practice.

There have also been important policy changes. There is an increasingly widespread call for patient and public involvement in all aspects of health and social care, service provision and research. Policy initiatives and guidance documents from the Department of Health currently explicitly state that research studies should include input from consumers (DoH 1989, 1991, 1997, 1998a, 1998b, 1998c, 1999a, 1999b, 2000a, 2000b, 2001a, 2001b, 2001c; NHS Executive 1996; NHS Executive et al. 1998).

Specific developments within cancer

In the field of cancer, involving patients in the research process has, in the past, been limited compared with other diseases. The publication of the Calman-Hine Report (DoH 1995) was a key watershed in terms of establishing the principles that cancer services should be patient centred and incorporate wider community perspectives. Consumer involvement received specific endorsement in the *NHS Cancer Plan* published in 2000, and in the *National Service Framework Assessments for Cancer Care* published in 2001. The *Report of the National Cancer Taskforce on User Involvement in Cancer Services* called for full integration of consumer involvement into Cancer Network structures at the national, regional and local levels (Bradburn 2001).

Following the Calman-Hine Report, 34 Cancer Networks were established. Each Network has its own specialist Cancer Centre and satellite Cancer Units. Cancer Research Networks were also created with the same geographical boundaries. A number of new national institutions were also created. The National Cancer Research Network (NCRN) was set up in 2001 to provide the necessary infrastructure and support for all the Research Networks, while the National Cancer Research Institute (NCRI) was formed in the same year to provide a strategic overview of cancer research. The National Translational Cancer Research Network (NTRAC) was formed in 2001 to speed the transference of results from the laboratory into routine care. The NCRN also co-ordinates 23 Clinical Studies Groups. The primary aim of each group is to develop new clinical studies and then take them forward for funding. They also provide expert advice, oversee existing studies and are linked to the NCRN and NTRAC. Individual groups exist for all of the principal tumour sites and there are a number of generic groups such as radiotherapy, palliative care, psychosocial oncology, primary care and complementary therapies. Each group brings together the leading UK experts, with consumers, in that particular specialty.

In 2003, a full-time Consumer Liaison Lead was appointed by the NCRN to support consumer involvement initiatives in cancer research. Key objectives include ensuring consumer representation in the NCRI Clinical Studies Groups, developing consumer involvement in research at local and regional levels within the Cancer Research Networks, fostering consumer involvement within the Clinical Trials Units and increasing public awareness about cancer research in general.

These changes and initiatives have presented many opportunities for consumer involvement within UK cancer research. In the following section, examples are provided of how consumer involvement is being incorporated into cancer research at all levels.

Examples of consumer involvement in action

Consumer involvement within the national organizations

There is increasing representation of consumers within other associated organizations. The Medical Research Council (MRC) established its own Consumer Liaison Group in March 2000 to advise on ways of promoting effective and appropriate consumer involvement in its activities and to ensure that the MRC is aware of, and able to respond to, consumer interests and concerns about research. A consumer was also appointed in 2003 to sit on the Clinical Trials Advisory and Awards Committee (CTAAC), the joint committee developed by the MRC and Cancer Research UK to streamline the peer review process of cancer trial proposals. Consumers have also been appointed as peer reviewers to the Cochrane Collaboration to comment on draft reviews and protocols (http://www.cochrane.de).

A survey of clinical trial co-ordinating centres (Hanley et al. 2001) reported that 23 out of 62 centres involved consumers and a further 17 centres planned to involve consumers. Respondents were generally positive about consumer involvement and said that it helped refine the research question, improved the quality of patient information and made the trial more relevant to patients' needs. Clinical Trials Units are now undergoing an accreditation process and are increasingly looking toward the involvement of consumers in their activities.

There is consumer representation on the NCRI Board and on the steering and subgroups, which guide NCRN and NTRAC. Consumers are also represented on the Strategic Planning Groups – for Supportive and Palliative Care, Prevention and Risk, and Radiotherapy and Radiobiology. In addition, there is consumer representation on the NCRI Clinical Trials Board Sub-Group and the NCRI Translational Research Board Sub-Group.

Derek Stewart is a former cancer patient who was a member of the Head and Neck and Radiotherapy Clinical Studies Groups. Derek was the first chair of the NCRI Consumer Liaison Group and as such a member of the NCRI Board before stepping down from this role in 2004. Derek writes:

> It is important to remember that the 'patient' was a person before diagnosis, with a wealth of transferable skills, knowledge and experience. 'Consumer involvement', in the context of the national cancer organizations, is the full and active participation with professionals to help improve research. The normal description of consumer involvement is often narrowed within the confines of the research cycle and referred to either as consultation, collaboration and/or consumer led. However in cancer research this has been broadened to include participation in the national strategic management, decision making, planning subgroups, peer review processes and awards committees. Our function, as patients taking a positive role in cancer research consumer involvement, is developing into one of active presence, vigilant watcher, contributor to the dialogue and challenging partner.
>
> As 'active presence', we have an expectation of being asked to participate, sitting at the table and acting as a physical reminder of the purpose.
>
> As 'vigilant watcher' we are able to witness that the patients' interests are being considered, but we must make sure that people continue working together and make maximum use of resources.
>
> As a 'contributor to the dialogue' it is about having a right to add our voice with a responsibility to gain an understanding of the issues.
>
> As a 'challenging partner' we may want to be involved in our own research, spending time listening to different patient communities and as a by-product becoming advocates for research in general.
>
> Using this model has significantly altered the notion of merely seeking views, and displays a much broader concept of participation. This illustrates commitment at the highest echelons, transparency of process and openness to procedures and is demonstrated by the extent of consumer involvement now taking place.

Professor Janet Darbyshire, director of the MRC Clinical Trials Unit, gives her own views about consumer involvement within national organizations:

> I first experienced the value of consumer involvement at all stages of the research process in the field of HIV/AIDS and learnt the importance of demonstrating its value to other researchers. From the early days of MRC trials in HIV/AIDS, consumers were involved in the strategic and oversight committees for clinical trials as well as the individual trial development groups and steering committees. I welcomed the opportunity to be involved since the earliest stages of the development of the NCRI Consumer Liaison Group (CLG). It is crucial that the CLG provides the opportunity for dialogue between researchers and consumers – although inevitably the members, both researchers and consumers, are likely to be those who are already committed to the concept. The importance of providing adequate support, training and mentoring for consumers to enable them to fully participate in discussions with confidence, cannot be underestimated and should be adequately resourced.

One of the strengths of the NCRN and NCRI is that we can ensure that the consumer input is in place at all levels from local networks through to trial steering committees and Clinical Studies Groups (CSGs). The CLG has a key role in co-ordinating and overseeing this activity and providing the opportunity for consumers and researchers to evaluate them together. The importance of evaluating the benefits and challenges of consumer involvement is widely acknowledged, as is the difficulty in undertaking such evaluation. It is important for members of the CLG and the CSGs to be involved in setting the parameters of these evaluations. Finally, decisions about turnover of membership, selection of new members and most important, the chair, also need to be considered in line with other CSGs, but taking into account the differences.

Consumer involvement within the NCRI Clinical Studies Groups

The NCRI Consumer Liaison Group was formed in June 2000 to provide a national overview of consumer concerns and act as a central resource for guidance on consumer issues. It develops and co-ordinates strategic partnerships across key organizations and provides advice and support to consumers and researchers. The majority of members are people who have direct experience of cancer as patients, family members or carers. Some are people who work in cancer research and support organizations. Most members are also consumer representatives on one of the NCRI Clinical Studies Groups. Two consumers sit on each group.

Some scientific knowledge is helpful but not necessary, as consumers bring to the groups an in-depth experience of their particular disease area. Consumers are asked to focus on three central questions:

* How will this research benefit the patient?
* Will the burden outweigh the benefit?
* What is the long-term gain for all patients?

The NCRN and NCRI believe that consumer input into the groups will help result in:

* improved recruitment, as studies that consumers have helped design may be studies that patients are more likely to enter.
* more patient centred study outcome measures, more valid and robust studies and wider ranging studies investigating research questions at all stages of the disease trajectory.
* a more balanced trials portfolio covering both standards of care and scientific innovations.

Ongoing evaluation of all NCRN and NCRI consumer involvement activity is designed to assess the impact on these markers.

David Kirby, a consumer who sits on the NCRI Upper Gastrointestinal (GI) Cancer Clinical Studies Group, presents an overview of his experiences:

As a survivor of oesophageal cancer and founder of the Oesophageal Patients Association (OPA), I was invited to join the Upper GI Clinical Studies Group of the

NCRI in 2001. From the outset in 1985, the OPA has worked closely with medical experts treating oesophageal cancer around the UK, aiming to be a responsible and knowledgeable group offering information of quality and sound guidance to patients and their carers on diagnosis of the disease.

The experience gained by this extensive contact with the medical teams is invaluable when joining a group of experts dealing with the scientific boundaries in this field. It also provides credibility within such a group, although the limits of one's knowledge are soon explored. However, the discussion at the group's meetings also demonstrates how much there is yet to learn which may possibly surprise the lay person. One finds, therefore, that involvement often means using a questioning technique, hopefully stimulating the thinking about an aspect. It is somewhat daunting attending the first meeting of the group – daunting but friendly.

Recently, a mentor has been nominated for the patient representative, a role I strongly advocate for any patient/carer group. It is important for the mentor to understand the motivation of the patient/carer in becoming involved. Obviously, this stems from the experience of the illness; the desire that all may survive; the desire that the effect of treatment on the patient's quality of life is understood and considered when delivered to patients at various stages of their illness and at various ages and attitudes to life; and their desire that treatments may become simpler, more predictable and universally available. Similarly, patients/carers are aware of the significant existence of secondary cancers not detected when treatment is begun and the effect this can have on the patient's quality of life.

Since the survival rate for upper GI cancers is poor, it may be that feedback from analysis of the work done by expert members of a Clinical Studies Group could be an influence on colleagues within the primary care field for earlier diagnosis, or even prevention.

I am informed that the presence of a patient/carer at such group meetings does influence the tenor of discussions particularly on quality of life aspects and this is gratifying. The patient/carer would thus like to see the expertise that is concentrated within the Clinical Studies Group having an influence on the earlier and later stages of the illness for the benefit of all.

Professor David Cunningham, chair of the NCRI Upper GI Cancer Clinical Studies Group, is supportive of consumer involvement at this level and writes:

The management of patients with upper gastrointestinal malignancy such as oesophageal cancer presents a real challenge. Overall survival in this particular patient group is poor and relapse following treatment is all too common. One of the major priorities for the Upper GI Cancer Clinical Studies Group is to improve this situation by identifying key research areas and facilitating the transition from valid research questions to robust clinical studies.

Intrinsic to this process is the valuable input from people whose lives have either been directly or indirectly affected by cancer. The integration of consumer perspective with expert opinion aids study selection and design and therefore potential patient recruitment, which is vital if the question posed by the study is to be answered accurately. Clinical endpoints help to define the importance of a study but without appropriate quality of life assessments, they become meaningless. The development of patient centred outcomes is paramount and only possible with consumer input and advice. As chair of the Upper GI Cancer Clinical Studies group, I feel it is valuable to have people like David Kirby as part of the group and fully support partnerships like this developing across the whole spectrum of cancer management.

Consumer involvement within the Cancer Research Networks

We have seen how, at a national level, a strategy for consumer involvement has evolved. Consumer involvement at the Research Network level is perhaps the most fundamental in terms of the opportunities available for individuals to exercise their influence and provide an input into the development of studies at the earliest possible stage. In this section, we shall describe a successful model of such consumer involvement.

As part of the organizational changes described earlier, the North Trent Cancer Research Network (NTCRN) was established. Based in Sheffield, it extends across four satellite Cancer Units in Barnsley, Chesterfield, Doncaster/Bassetlaw and Rotherham and has a catchment population of nearly 2 million people (see websites http://www.ncrn.org.uk/Networks/index.htm and http://www.shef.ac.uk/ntcrn/index. html).

In response to a growing need to incorporate more systematically the views of consumers in its research programme, the NTCRN allocated monies from its funds to set up a Consumer Research Panel (CRP). Researchers at the Academic Palliative Medicine Unit (APMU) at the University of Sheffield were asked to co-ordinate the formation of the panel. Most members were recruited from delegates attending the Cancer Research Open Day consumer conference, held in Sheffield in 2001. The panel consists of people who have experience of a range of cancers, as patients or carers, and who are interested in research. A database of members' interests and abilities facilitates the most suitable channels for individual input and expression. Advice was sought from other bodies, including research ethics committees, which also seek to include the views and opinions of lay members, in order that appropriate terms of reference were developed. There are two co-chairs, both of whom are cancer patients.

Training is a key element in successful consumer involvement and enhancing an individual's capacity to participate. Unfamiliarity with structures, processes and terminology can be daunting. To ensure that members feel equipped to engage with the research community, a two-day introductory training course and a mentoring scheme has been established. Ongoing evaluation of the training programme remains very positive.

NTCRN panel members are reimbursed for their time, in addition to their travel and subsistence expenses. These costs are met directly from each of the projects or groups that request consumer representation. The panel is supported by the APMU, through a research fellow, Dr Karen Collins, and a secretary, Mrs Sue Button.

Since the advent of the Consumer Research Panel, consumers in North Trent have had the opportunity to influence the research agenda at all stages of the process and in diverse ways. Members have taken part in advisory groups offering their views on studies in the developmental stage. Groups have been set up for proposed projects investigating the use of thalidomide in cachectic patients and a study examining artificial hydration in terminally ill patients (Ahmedzai et al. 2004). Panel members are regular attendees at Cancer Research Network and cancer project board meetings, and on project steering groups.

Consumers have presented papers at local, regional and national conferences. Consumers are assisting in analysis and dissemination and have contributed to publications (Stevens et al. 2003a, 2003b; Wilde et al. 2003). In all of these ventures, newer members are helped and guided by more experienced mentors and no consumer attends an event without either the support of a fellow member or a researcher who is experienced in working with consumers. This kind of mentoring scheme has been used successfully elsewhere (Consumer Involvement in HTA Research 2000).

For the NTCRN, consumer involvement is a performance indicator in its Network Plan. The Network has recognized the value of the CRP and in 2004, more than doubled the funding available to the panel for the next financial year. This will enable the panel to increase its membership and thus to make itself available to more researchers across the Network.

Dawn Wragg, co-chair of the NTCRN Consumer Research Panel, provides a consumer's perspective of what it means to be involved in the field of cancer research:

> I was 31 years old when I was told I had breast cancer. I felt an urgent need to reassess my life and think very carefully about what I still needed to achieve. During this process I made a conscious decision to use my experiences in a positive way, wanting to give something back and make a difference while getting back some form of control over my life – common feelings for someone with a life-threatening illness. I received a letter through the post inviting me to attend a meeting regarding a new group being piloted in Sheffield that gave consumers the opportunity to contribute to and influence cancer research. The group appeared to have very firm foundations with clear support structures and very specific roles. Induction was thorough, giving valuable advice and building confidence. I was particularly impressed by the very strong feeling that the group would not be tokenistic – there was a genuine feeling of need and value for consumer involvement. I felt this was the perfect opportunity for me to use my skills and experiences in a positive way. I joined the panel and was eventually elected co-chair.
>
> Panel members are encouraged to work in pairs in order to share the workload, build confidence and for general reassurance in a new and sometimes daunting arena. As co-chair I feel it is essential to support and encourage members to participate where they see an opportunity to do so and identify necessary training needs so they feel confident and equipped to help. Our greatest responsibility is to ensure that challenges to consumer involvement are removed.
>
> As a member of the panel I have been involved in analysing qualitative research data, the results of which have now been published (Stevens et al. 2003b) and we are currently working on a follow-up paper. I was welcomed into this team of professionals giving me the confidence to share my views, providing a patient's perspective and having some influence on the final outcome. I now represent the panel on the NTCRN Project Board and at the Clinical Trials Executive which gives me the opportunity to be involved at a more strategic level. The panel also organizes an annual consumer conference that attracts highly regarded speakers discussing current topics chosen by consumers.
>
> I feel my involvement has given me the opportunity to do something positive with my experiences, hopefully helping others and influencing change in a very small way.

However, I appreciate that there are still some challenges facing consumer involvement. How do we ensure diverse representation? Can one person who has experience of one type of cancer represent the views of their peers? How does one prevent a consumer with a personal issue using this forum for their own problems? And should one try? Consumers can be overwhelmed by unrealistic expectations with no allowances made for their fatigue, or the amount of time they can actually give. Balancing the difference between a 'professional patient' and a patient who acts professionally may be difficult. In my experience, I have found that patience, time, training, and educating professionals are all ways to help address these issues. The greatest challenge of all is inadequate resources. Without stable funding or dedicated time, it is impossible to provide satisfactory support and encourage development.

Monitoring and evaluation of the panel has shown that a structured, well supported group not only provides a stronger voice collectively but also builds the confidence of the participating individuals (Wilde et al. 2003). The considerable achievement of the panel highlights the advantages of a stable, valued group who will evolve with proper financial and time investment for the mutual benefit of consumers and professionals.

Professor Sam H. Ahmedzai, chair of the Academic Palliative Medicine Unit – which hosts the North Trent Cancer Research Network Consumer Research Panel – at the University of Sheffield, writes:

At first sight it might seem strange for a university unit of palliative medicine to be hosting a cancer network Consumer Research Panel. This relationship is explained through this unit's long-standing commitment to supportive care – a wide range of multidisciplinary interventions aimed at improving patient and carer well-being and functioning from the time of diagnosis. Arising from this interest, we initially became involved in research studies of newly diagnosed patients with breast, lung and colorectal cancer, which were examining their attitudes to participation in – or rejection of – cancer clinical trials.

Our engagement with cancer patients and their carers confirmed to us that we needed to give them a greater voice in the shape of cancer research itself. Thus, with the combined drive of key researchers such as Tony Stevens, David Wilde, Nisar Ahmed and John Hunt, we convinced the North Trent Cancer Research Network to fund a trial year of a new venture – the Consumer Research Panel. The success of that has been described above and was underlined by the increased financial commitment shown by the North Trent Cancer Research Network in 2004.

What are the main lessons I have learnt from working with consumers in the panel? First, it has become clearer to me that cancer patients and their carers have valuable insights into the symptom and psychosocial burden of cancer and its treatments – and they are better than any professional at expressing the impact of this in their daily lives. Second, my colleagues in the academic unit and I have learnt that if we can't explain a research proposal in everyday language that consumers can understand, then we need to go back and clarify our own thoughts about the work. Third, I have been excited by the experience of working alongside consumers as advisers, co-researchers and co-authors on research papers, which makes the research much more 'real' and 'live' compared to the standard way of conducting research on consumers.

Challenges in consumer involvement

What has been addressed?

A number of significant challenges that have previously constrained consumer involvement have been overcome. These include issues of recruitment and representation, payments to consumers, developing collaborative relationships between consumers and members of the research community, providing appropriate training, education and mentoring, and establishing working relationships with other cancer research organizations.

First, regarding recruitment and representation, there has been considerable success in recruiting consumers at a national level and the example of a Consumer Research Panel based in North Trent indicates some of the ways that consumers are being involved within the Cancer Research Networks. These developments have been the result of careful attention being paid to the issues of constituency (the individuals or groups being represented) and authority (who is the representative). The examples of involvement outlined here have been founded upon a broad-based recruitment strategy. Thus, there is scope for input from individuals (including family members and carers), who can draw on their personal experiences, as outlined by Entwistle et al. (1998), as well as representatives from national charities and consumer groups, and consumer advocates who are able to synthesize and articulate the views of others. The question of representation is often a recurrent, but essentially redundant, criticism of consumer involvement – it is unlikely that any group or organization could be said to be truly representative.

Some progress has been made toward the greater involvement of consumers from black and ethnic minority population groups. In 2001, the National Cancer Alliance collaborated with consumers from several different ethnic backgrounds on a study to adapt their 'Teamwork File' for use by people from black and ethnic minority groups, and other socially disadvantaged groups, in Oxford, Leicester and Birmingham (National Cancer Alliance 2002). Consumers were active in prioritizing topic areas, planning, managing and designing the research, analysing the data and implementing the resulting actions. However, at all levels, additional efforts are required to increase the involvement of certain groups – for example, those patients with a poor prognosis and those with a good prognosis, older and younger consumers, as well as individuals from black and ethnic minority groups.

Second, the issue of payments to consumers has been addressed. All consumers who take part in NCRN and NCRI activities are reimbursed for their input in accordance with current good practice (Steel 2003). In addition, travel and other expenses are covered and a resource fund exists to cover other outlays, for example, costs of caring for dependent family members. However, local arrangements within Research Networks need to be developed to ensure an element of uniformity (Wilde et al. 2003).

Third, the efforts to develop a collaborative working relationship between consumers and the research community have been successful. It has been said that consumers, with no formal training in medicine or research methods will be able to give only a non-scientific, partial view clouded by their own subjective experiences. Some professionals have argued that patients may generalise from their own individual, highly variable experiences, which is completely counter to the medico-scientific paradigm of knowledge development (Canter 2001). This situation may be exacerbated if there is a lack of clarity in the dialogue with consumers about their role. On the one hand, consumers may feel that it is not necessary to understand the underlying science of a research study, as their presence is to provide the patient perspective. On the other hand, consumers may feel there are prohibitions about speaking from their own personal experience (Tranter and Sullivan 1996), when in fact, this is one of the strengths of consumer input. Health professional and consumer members of the Clinical Studies Groups are committed to understanding the perspective of others and this has been a crucial factor in establishing effective working relationships, as other research has indicated (Oliver et al. 2001). Evaluation of consumer representation at group meetings indicates that a truly collaborative relationship is developing between all Clinical Studies Group members. Within the NTCRN, similar monitoring processes exist and other Research Networks will be able to adapt these.

Fourth, an important issue that has been addressed is the provision of support to consumer representatives. Nationally, within the NCRN and NCRI, and at Research Network level within the NTCRN, induction programmes have been developed to:

- Familiarize representatives with the organization of the cancer research community
- provide some background information about clinical trials and other kinds of research
- facilitate effective consumer input into meetings.

Two consumers are represented on all NCRN and NCRI activities, which in addition to providing mutual support, helps maintain continuity of input and a broader perspective. Each consumer has access to a scientific mentor, who is available before meetings to clarify any issues, to be present during meetings to provide support and be accessible after meetings for feedback. There is ongoing support, training and education based on the results of an annual training assessment questionnaire. In addition, consumers can access training courses for Cancer Research Network staff. Consumers are also encouraged to attend national conferences and meetings that are appropriate to their specialist interests. Consumer representatives also have free access to academic libraries and electronic journals.

The other major issue that is being tackled is fostering co-operation between different national and regional organizations and the cancer charities. There are several logistical challenges that need to be addressed when supporting a relatively small, geographically spread group of consumers. For example, there can be limited scope to take advantage of economies of scale, which can increase the costs of the delivery of training. Attention is focusing on working with other organizations to minimize duplication and reduce costs. In addition, the possibilities afforded by innovative applications of information technology are being explored, such as video-conferencing, email distribution list, web forums and support groups, downloadable multimedia and access to virtual professionals (Street 2003).

The NCRN is also working with Macmillan Cancer Relief on a jointly funded initiative to ensure that all Cancer Research Networks will be able to support consumer involvement in research at a local and regional level.

What issues remain to be addressed?

Despite the real advances that have been made, a number of challenges remain. A priority must be to increase and broaden the involvement of consumers from black and ethnic minorities. Equally, attention needs to focus upon the involvement and inclusion of patients from poor prognosis groups. Some work has been carried out by researchers, carers and palliative care patients at the Worthing and Southlands Hospitals NHS Trust to find out what service users want from a palliative care service (INVOLVE Project Database Title 4 2001–3). Engaging with isolated individuals (both geographically and socially), older consumers and younger consumers are also important. Using information and communications technology in innovative ways may be one route for facilitating this.

The involvement of consumers in research priority setting exercises has been limited in the past. However, consumers on the Clinical Studies Groups now have the opportunity to influence this area. In 2003, Macmillan Cancer Relief began a series of consultation exercises with consumers to ascertain their research priorities. Macmillan has stated that the results of these consultations will be used to inform their organization's research agenda.

Greater efforts need to be made to involve consumers in dissemination, for example, improving access to results, increasing consumer activity in actual dissemination and improving the clarity of reporting of findings. There is a need to encourage more user led research, particularly in the evaluation of consumer involvement activity. Organizations such as Folk.Us (http://latis.ex.ac.uk/folk.us) have demonstrated that consumers can conduct robust studies in this field. Nationally, clarification of the impact of payments upon those in receipt of benefits is an issue that requires urgent attention. Standardizing reimbursement processes for consumers is a challenge that remains at Research Network level.

Developing accessible training, education, mentoring and support opportunities at all levels and stages of the research process remains an ongoing task. The joint Macmillan Cancer Relief/National Cancer Research Network project referred to earlier aims to develop a portfolio of training that is freely accessible. A similar resource has already been created in Australia at the National Resource Centre for Consumer Participation in Health, co-ordinated through La Trobe University (http://www.participateinhealth.org.au).

Involving consumers in strategies to increase public awareness of medical research is also a significant area of work. There is evidence that low awareness of research is an important factor in affecting accrual to randomized trials (Stevens and Ahmedzai 2004). Consumer representatives are working with Macmillan Cancer Relief, NTRAC and Sir Iain Chalmers, from the James Lind Initiative, to raise public awareness in this area. Consumers and representatives from NCRN are also collaborating with Consumer for Ethics in Research (http://www.ceres.org.uk) to establish and evaluate an independent information and advice service to provide support for potential and existing participants in medical research.

Finally, the identification of sustainable funding streams for consumer involvement activity remains an important issue both nationally and locally. The collation of evidence of successful consumer involvement activity will help secure future funding bids. To do this, the involvement of consumers and their collaboration with research teams must be carefully and consistently documented from the inception of a study to its completion and evaluation.

Conclusion

The movement to involve consumers in cancer research has grown rapidly since the early 1990s. Some general observations can be drawn about the level and nature of this involvement. In order that consumers are able to exercise their influence appropriately, there needs to be clarity about accountability and the constituencies consumers are able to represent.

Initiatives should also be inclusive and involve hard to reach and vulnerable groups. Consumer activities need to be integrated with existing community and voluntary networks to minimize duplication. At the same time, consumers should feel confident that they are able to articulate their views independently, and in a way that promotes shared decision making rather than tokenism. Identification of ongoing funding streams to support this activity is essential to support payments to consumers, expenses and training. Within cancer, many of these issues have been successfully addressed.

Perhaps the major challenge remaining is that of evaluation. The aforementioned NTCRN Consumer Research Panel has been positively evaluated by the University of Sheffield's School of Health and Related Research (Cooper 2004). However, there remains a paucity of evaluative studies that have examined whether the involvement of consumers has had any significant effect on patient outcomes. Although some progress has been made (Tritter et al. 2003), the evaluation of consumer involvement in research remains intrinsically difficult – primarily because of a lack of any consensus in defining outcome measures. The authors would strongly recommend that all activities involving consumers in research should have a strong evaluative component. There is an urgent need for consumers themselves need to engage in this debate and be involved in thorough and robust evaluations that can explore both processes and outcomes of consumer involvement in research activity.

Cancer is one of the first diseases to have offered real opportunities for consumers to influence research by promoting consumer representation at national, regional and local levels. The formation of a new infrastructure to support research activity and provide a strategic overview of cancer research is providing a unique opportunity to integrate and extend the scope of consumer involvement at national and Research Network levels. Elements of the model of involvement that has been successfully developed within cancer could be implemented in other diseases and other health care settings.

Bibliography

Ahmedzai, S.H., Wilman, K., Wragg, D., Paz, S. and Hillam, S. (2004) 'Engaging consumers on ethical issues in palliative care research', *Palliative Medicine*, 18: 168.

Bradburn, J. (2001) *Report of the National Cancer Taskforce on User Involvement in Cancer Services*, London: National Cancer Taskforce.

Canter, R. (2001) 'Patients and medical power', *British Medical Journal*, 323: 414.

Consumer Involvement in HTA Research (2000) *Consumer Involvement in the Health*

Technology Assessment Programme, Southampton: National Coordinating Centre for Health Technology Assessment.

Cooper, C. (2004) 'An evaluation of the North Trent Cancer Research Network Consumer Research Panel', Sheffield: University of Sheffield, School of Health and Related Research.

Department of Health (1989) *NHS and Community Care Act*, London: HMSO.

Department of Health (1991) *The Patient's Charter*, London: HMSO.

Department of Health (1995) *A Policy Framework for Commissioning Cancer Services: A Report of the Expert Advisory Group on Cancer to the Chief Medical Officers of England and Wales (Calman-Hine Report)*, London: DoH.

Department of Health (1997) *The New NHS: Modern and Dependable*, London: The Stationery Office.

Department of Health (1998a) *A First Class Service*, London: The Stationery Office.

Department of Health (1998b) *Our Healthier Nation: A Contract for Health*, London: The Stationery Office.

Department of Health (1998c) *Health in Partnership: Patient, Carer and Public Involvement in Health Care Decision Making*, London: DoH.

Department of Health (1999a) *Patient and Public Involvement in the New NHS*, London: DoH.

Department of Health (1999b) *Making a Difference: Strengthening the Nursing, Midwifery and Health Visiting Contribution to Health and Health Care*, London: DoH.

Department of Health (2000a) *The NHS Plan: A Plan for Investment, A Plan for Reform*, London: The Stationery Office.

Department of Health (2000b) *Needs of the Patients Top the New NHS Agenda: National Health Service News, Summer*, Leeds: NHS Executive and DoH.

Department of Health (2001a) *The Essence of Care: Patient-focused Benchmarking for Health Care Practitioners*, London: DoH.

Department of Health (2001b) *The Expert Patient: A New Approach to Chronic Disease Management for the 21st Century*, London: DoH.

Department of Health (2001c) *The Report of the Public Inquiry into Children's Heart Surgery at the Bristol Royal Infirmary, 1984–95: Learning the Lessons from Bristol*, London: DoH.

Entwistle, V.A., Renfrew, M.J., Yearley, S., Forester, J. and Lamont, T. (1998) 'Lay perspectives: advantages for health research', *British Medical Journal*, 316: 463–6.

Goodare, H. and Smith, R. (1995) 'The rights of patients in research', *British Medical Journal*, 310: 1277–8.

Guadagnoli, E. and Ward, P. (1998) 'Patient participation in decision making', *Social Science and Medicine*, 47: 329–39.

Hanley, B., Truesdale, A., King, A., Elbourne, D. and Chalmers, I. (2001) 'Involving consumers in designing, conducting and interpreting randomised controlled trials: questionnaire survey', *British Medical Journal*, 322: 519–23.

INVOLVE Project Database Title 4 (2001–3) *An Exploration of What Service Users Want and Experience from Palliative Care: A Participatory Study* (available http://www.invo.org.uk/pub.htm).

National Cancer Alliance (2002) *Information Needs of South Asian Cancer Patients and Carers: A Qualitative Study*, Oxford: National Cancer Alliance.

National Cancer Research Institute (NCRI) (2002) *Strategic Analysis*, London: NCRI.

NHS Executive (1996) *Patient Partnership: Building a Collaborative Strategy*, Leeds: NHS Executive.

NHS Executive, Institute of Health Services Management and NHS Confederation (1998) *In the Public Interest: Developing a Strategy for Public Participation in the NHS*, Leeds: NHS Executive Quality and Consumers Branch.

Oliver, S.R., Milne, R., Bradburn, J., Buchanan, P., Kerridge, L., Walley, T. and Gabbay, J. (2001) 'Involving consumers in a needs-led research programme: a pilot project', *Health Expectations*, 4: 18–28.

Ong, B.N. (1996) 'The lay perspective in health technology assessment, *International Journal of Technology Assessment in Health Care*, 12: 511–17.

Steel, R. (2003) *A Guide to Paying Members of the Public who are Actively Involved in Research*, 2nd Edn, Eastleigh, Hampshire: INVOLVE.

Stevens, T. and Ahmedzai, S.H. (2004) 'Why do breast cancer patients decline randomised trials of adjuvant therapy and what do they think about their decision later?', *Patient Education and Counselling*, 52 (3): 341–8.

Stevens, T., Wilde, D., Hunt, J. and Ahmedzai, S.H. (2003a) 'Overcoming the challenges to consumer involvement in cancer research', *Health Expectations*, 6: 81–8.

Stevens, T., Wilde, D., Paz, S., Rawson, A., Wragg, D. and Ahmedzai, S.H. (2003b) 'Palliative care research protocols: a special case for ethical review?', *Palliative Medicine*, 17: 482–90.

Street Jr, R.L. (2003) 'Mediated consumer-provider communication in cancer care: the empowering potential of new technologies', *Patient Education and Counselling*, 50: 99–104

Tranter, G. and Sullivan, S. (1996) 'Whose shout?', *Health Service Journal*, 2: 31.

Tritter, J., Daykin, N., Evans, S. and Sanidas, M. (2003) *Improving Cancer Services through Patient Involvement*, Oxford: Radcliffe.

Wanless, D. (2002) *Securing our Future Health: Taking a Long-Term View*, London: HM Treasury.

Wilde, D., Collins, K., Stevens, T., Hunt, J., Button, S. and Ahmedzai, S.H. (2003) *The North Trent Cancer Research Network Consumer Research Panel: Annual Review*, Annual Report, Sheffield: North Trent Cancer Research Network.

Further reading

Boote, J., Telford, R. and Cooper, C. (2002) 'Consumer involvement in health research: a review and research agenda', *Health Policy*, 61: 213–26.

Gott, M., Stevens, T., Small, N. and Ahmedzai, S.H. (2002) 'Involving users, improving services: the example of cancer', *British Journal of Clinical Governance*, 7: 81–5.

Hanley, B., Bradburn, J., Barnes, M., Evans, C., Goodare, H., Kelson, M., Kent, A., Oliver, S., Thomas, S. and Wallcraft, J. (2003) *Involving the Public in NHS, Public Health, and Social Care Research: Briefing Notes for Researchers*, 2nd Edn, Eastleigh, Hampshire: INVOLVE.

Small, N. and Rhodes, P. (2000) *Too Ill to Talk? User Involvement and Palliative Care*, London: Routledge.

Stevens, T., Wilde, D., Hunt, J. and Ahmedzai, S.H. (2003) 'Overcoming the challenges to consumer involvement in cancer research', *Health Expectations*, 6: 81–8.

Thornton, H. (2002) 'Patient perspectives on involvement in cancer research in the UK', *European Journal of Cancer Care*, 11: 205–9.

Chapter 10

Community action to housing and health research

Meryl Basham with Diane Stockton and
Michelle Lake on behalf of the Torbay Healthy Housing Group

Introduction

Involving the public in health research has gained credence in recent years through the work of the Consumers in NHS Research, now renamed INVOLVE. Several key influential documents have been published including, 'Involving consumers in designing, conducting, and interpreting randomized controlled trials: questionnaire survey' (Hanley et al. 2001) and 'Involving consumers in research and development in the NHS: briefing notes for researchers' (Hanley et al. 2000). In April 2001, the role of Consumers in NHS Research expanded to include public health and social care research outside of the NHS, giving a broad base of potential influences on the prioritizing of research. Housing and health research is a public health issue particularly for those most vulnerable, such as elderly people, the very young or those with a disability (Department of Health 2001; British Medical Association 2003).

Randomized controlled trials are still regarded as the most methodologically rigorous method of assessing health care interventions. However, the degree of participation in research projects varies considerably, on a continuum of being totally controlled by professionals to being totally led by the public. This is particularly so in clinical randomized controlled trials, and there is little published hard data about the extent or impact of public involvement in housing and health research (Consumers in NHS Research et al. 2000; Crawford et al. 2002).

We describe here the pathway of community involvement, which led to a randomized controlled trial in housing and health, the Watcombe Housing Project (Somerville et al. 2002), and the impact of tenants' involvement upon the house improvement and research process. Tenants or 'local people' in social housing are the terms generally used to describe study participants.

Watcombe Housing Project

The origins of the project arose from a family GP voicing his concerns to the locality manager of primary care (at that time) about the high number of visits and call outs to his practice, which were mainly the areas of Barton, Watcombe and Hele in the seaside resort of Torquay in South Devon. A community consultation resulted, held at a local pub, with over 50 people attending including local people, councillors and statutory and voluntary organizations. The report from this event (Gay 1994) indicated that at that time, using the Jarman index for deprivation, the population of these areas was 22.7 compared with the Devon average of 12.75.

Following the report's recommendations, a three-year health gain initiative project, using community development methods, was funded from 1995 to 1998 by the then South and West Devon Health Authority. Three tenants were elected (at an open community event) as representatives of local people, one from each of the areas of Barton, Watcombe and Hele, to sit on the multi-agency steering committee of the project. The Initiative published several local reports (Barton, Watcombe and Hele Health Gain Initiative 1998).

Community survey

Social housing tenants in Watcombe expressed their concerns, about damp and condensation in their houses and the incidence of children's asthma, to their representative on the Health Gain Initiative, who subsequently put forward the suggestion of a survey of households, to find out the extent of the problems. With the support of the community worker and Dr Hilary Neve (adviser to the project), a questionnaire survey was devised to assess the perceived problems in this clearly defined area of council rented accommodation. A pictorial guide drawn by one of the tenants was used to define condensation/damp and mould. Local people, who volunteered to do the interviews, were given nominal expenses and received informal training about interview techniques and personal safety; 96 households were interviewed during the winter of 1996. The results were collated into a report that indicated that dampness was self-reported by 64 per cent of tenants and that 56 per cent (47/84) reported a health problem, the most common being asthma (Basham and Neve 1997). Although some questionnaires were incomplete, the community survey did give a clearer indication of the extent of damp in houses and the health of tenants.

Moving forward

With the support of the Health Gain Initiative, an extended inter-agency steering group (including the tenant representative and an adviser from the Plymouth and South Devon Research and Development Support Unit) formed the Torbay Healthy Housing Group. Following much lobbying by the group, agreement was gained in 1998 from the Council Housing Committee that £600,000 of the maintenance budget would be allocated to improve the houses in two phases, one year apart. The research questionnaires, interviews and environmental testing were completed over three years. Funding was obtained from the regional NHS Research and Development Committee to evaluate the proposed improvements, and the randomized controlled trial of the Watcombe Housing Project began in 1998. The community worker was appointed as research co-ordinator, providing a continuous link with tenants and agencies. The research question was 'Do house improvements influence the indoor environment, the health of tenants and costs to the NHS?'

Although changing over time, usually two local people represented study participants on the steering group throughout the three-year project. The relationships already established, during the community project, helped to ensure good communication and tenants were continually consulted, through newsletters, exhibitions and social events. All the literature used in the project was discussed with the representatives and amended if required to ensure readability.

Randomization

Opinions of local people varied regarding whose houses should be improved in the first phase, some feeling strongly that it should be those with ill health or small children while others felt it should be houses with no heating. The baseline survey of the study population indicated that ill health was spread across the area, so that to select people by specific need could have been perceived to be unfair. Randomization was explained by newsletter, posters in the local housing office on the estate, and face-to-face contact, which was the method seen to be most acceptable in research terms. It was perceived by tenants as being similar to a lottery, in that everyone had a chance of being chosen to be in the first phase. Following consultation, randomization took place in an unusual way, i.e. at a public meeting in a community room on the housing estate, with a local councillor picking the numbers of houses (first phase of 50 houses) out of a bucket, the remainder being allocated to the second phase of improvement the following year. Selection included a percentage of houses in each of the five streets of the area.

Participation in the research was high. In the first year, 119 households (n = 509 people) participated, with only 8 households refusing to take part. Evaluation included postal questionnaires to identify demographic and health details, and environmental testing of houses completed in January/February annually for three years. Health interviews, undertaken by community nurses, for specific illnesses of asthma, arthritis/rheumatism and angina and general health questionnaires were undertaken each May/June. High participation in the study continued throughout, although fewer health interviews were completed in the last year, feedback from tenants indicating that this was mainly due to questionnaire fatigue.

Structure of the project

The main multi-agency steering group had two subgroups: Health and Environment for the research element, and Housing for the improvement process. Tenant representatives were not part of the research subgroups, as they did not wish to be overloaded with frequent meetings, both having family commitments. However, consultation before meetings ensured that their viewpoint was aired on issues to be discussed. The key issue for tenants was improving their homes and their quality of life with the research being secondary. Molyneux (2003) suggests that it is a good idea to reflect about whether the issues or problems that encouraged someone to get involved in research in the first place were being addressed and certainly, parents of children suffering from asthma appeared to be motivated by that factor.

Tenant involvement and collaboration in the research process was extensive, including how the data were collected. However, their influence on the methods of outcomes measures was minimal. Most of these decisions were made when the funding protocol was written and validated questionnaires chosen to provide the robustness that was expected of a randomized controlled trial.

There were concerns, voiced by local people and health interviewers, about the research methods used, e.g. the General Health Questionnaire (GHQ12) used in the health interviews, with some people feeling uncomfortable about answering questions about mental health and what were perceived by tenants to be personal issues. The use of the GHQ12 and the SF36 (another general health questionnaire) was driven by the validity and current credibility given to them by the research establishment, and it was for these reasons that the research team decided that the questionnaires could not be changed.

Representation by the research team, including the tenant representatives, in the Housing subgroup was nil, but this was also the case for the Council Housing Department in the Health and Environmental subgroups. This caused difficulties with communication, such as lack of understanding of the importance of the renovation and research taking place at the same time each year and delays in contract work. However, the research process was discussed and sanctioned at the main steering group meetings and each subgroup reported to the steering group on a regular basis. Although a site presence by the Housing Department was assured at a regular time each week to deal with tenants' queries or difficulties, this rarely occurred, with visits being made ad hoc. This was reported by tenants to cause a great deal of frustration, as response to complaints was slow.

Role of the tenant (study participants) representatives

The role of the tenant representatives was key to the process, as they had regular contact with and gained information from other study participants, which was not always accessible to the research co-ordinator. Changes to the process of house improvements were instigated as a result of the tenant representatives' work, for example, a survey of the study houses found that there were problems with the ventilation fans installed during the renovation process. The fans were important both to householders and the research, as indoor air quality and the environment could have been affected, influencing the research outcomes. The survey highlighted that the fans were working unsatisfactorily and that there were additional problems with some contractors' attitudes, suggesting that as council tenants 'they had to accept what they were told', regarding the house improvements. Following presentation of the findings to the steering group, the fans were replaced or repaired by the Housing Department, which also inserted a clause into contracts for the following improvement phase, which indicated that respectful behaviour to tenants and their homes was expected. However, complaints about the quality of some contractors' work continued throughout the study, with residents feeling that they had little or no influence in the improvements to their homes. An example of this concerned the excessive use of trunking (wires covered by white plastic tubing instead of being chased into the wall) by some contractors, which some people were confident enough to challenge and, consequently, successfully influence what happened in their homes. Others who felt unable to do this were dissatisfied, and reported that the trunking 'looks like spaghetti on the wall'. Clearly, this method of wiring was for the contractors' convenience both in time and work, rather than for the satisfaction of the tenants.

An improvement to the research process, instigated by the tenant representatives, concerned advice about the way data were collected, thus appointments were made with householders for the environmental testing of their houses and health interviews. Local knowledge and experience in the community project had already shown that there was a reluctance to share information in public and attend public meetings. Interviews, therefore, took place in people's homes. This was more convenient for tenants, and feedback indicated that it had encouraged higher participation. This was confirmed by the generally high response rate.

We were fortunate in this study that the tenant representatives gave a great deal of their time freely, and were very committed to their role throughout the three years of the project. The involvement of study participants and the tenants' representatives in disseminating information about the study was extensive and included two videos. One, a housing studies training video (University of Bristol 2000) and the other, about involvement of tenants in the project, which was subsequently used in a conference presentation (Somerville et al. 2001). Two of the longest serving members, Diane Stockton and Michele Lake took part in various seminars about consumer involvement (Stockton and Basham 2002), participated in research telephone interviews and contributed to articles (Basham 2002). Both played a leading role in organizing community events, such as public meetings and Christmas parties, with even the research manager joining in as Father Christmas. The final community event they helped to organize was held at the local school, involving pupils, study participants and the public, to give feedback about the project results, and included demonstrations and activities about healthy lifestyles and energy efficiency.

Conclusion

There are examples of research that have been proactive in involving the public in the research process, but generally it is professionally led with little public involvement and collaboration, as outlined by Folk.Us, an organization in the forefront of promoting public involvement in research (Baxter et al. 2001). The Watcombe Project combined a public led approach to identifying the problem, i.e. the community survey initiated by local people, to 'professional led collaborative' where the involvement of tenants was under prescribed conditions. A key learning point is that the knowledge and experience of local people, living in the area, should be given equal value to that of researchers and housing managers.

The impact of the lack of personal control in regeneration and house improvement projects has been described as having a negative effect on people's health and lives (Allen 2000). The public often have low expectations of being involved, based on previous experience, resulting in the process being perceived as a professionalization of their neighbourhood's social problems, and their views tending to be valued only if they fitted in with others' interests (Elliott et al. 2001; Consumers in NHS Research et al. 2000). The tenant representatives in this project, at times, expressed feeling marginalized by the professionals involved in the research, but particularly with regard to decisions that were made about the house improvements. Comments included: 'people should be treated as individuals, with control over what happens in *their* house, as they pay the rent and have tenants' rights'. This experience was not unique, as other researchers have reported that people involved in house improvements expressed similar concerns and felt that the security that they had taken for granted could be threatened, and their individual wishes overridden (Elliott et al. 2001). As one tenant said, 'It's not just a house it's your home, [others should have] respect for people's homes'. More involvement by tenants both before and during the renovation process in this project would have been beneficial to help ensure tenant satisfaction.

There is an argument that the questions asked in research are ones the researchers wish to have answered and not the consumer (Consumers in NHS Research et al. 2000). Involving the public in designing the questions to be asked, and/or combined with using their own experiences in qualitative research, could enable more relevant research data. This was evidenced in the Watcombe Project, when the qualitative research interviews of a small sample of study participants identified negative and positive psycho-social effects, before and after the central heating was installed, which were not reflected by the validated questionnaires responses (Basham 2001).

To summarize tenant representatives' views of what had gone well from their point of view

- Having appointments for environmental testing and health interviews showed respect for people.
- Newsletters were important to provide regular information to tenants.
- The survey of tenants to enable action on unsatisfactory housing improvements was positive.
- Publicizing experience of public consultation through presentations at conferences is a valuable learning tool for others involved in housing improvement projects.

What could be improved

- Tenants should be consulted and involved from the beginning in the house improvement process, with individual householders being consulted and listened to by contractors regarding what occurs in their house.
- Contractors should be more accountable for their work and compensation given to tenants if the results are unsatisfactory.
- A questionnaire relating to the improvements, and tenants' satisfaction with them, should be completed before payment of contractors, as is usual in the private sector tenants should be involved in the improvement planning process and research protocol.
- On-site management could help with dealing with complaints more quickly.

It takes time to form collaborating partnerships and understanding of each other's priorities, which do not always coincide. To involve the public in research projects entails taking account of accessibility of meeting times, child-care and venue, language used and valuing the contribution they can make. Their contribution can be key to the success or otherwise of partnerships, and collaboration and consultation needs to begin at the planning stage of any housing improvement initiative.

References

Allen, T. (2000) 'Housing renewal – doesn't it make you sick?', *Housing Studies*, 15 (3): 443–61.

Barton, Watcombe and Hele Health Gain Initiative (1998) *Evaluation Report: Identifying Lessons Learned, Planning for Real, Community Report, and Parenting a Sound Investment for Torbay*, Torquay, Devon: Barton, Watcombe and Hele Health Gain Initiative.

Basham, M. (2001) 'Central heating – its influence on the use of the house, the behaviour and relationships of the household in wintertime', unpublished MSc dissertation, University of Plymouth.

Basham, M. (on behalf of the Torbay Healthy Housing Group) (2002) 'Community action to housing and health research', *Consumers in NHS Research Support Unit*, newsletter, Hampshire.

Basham, M. and Neve, H. (1997) *Watcombe Community Housing Survey*, Torquay, Devon: Barton, Watcombe and Hele Health Gain Initiative.

Baxter, L., Thorne, L. and Mitchell, A. (2001) *Small Voices, Big Noises: Lay Involvement in Health Research – Lessons from Other Fields*, Report by Folk.Us for Consumers in NHS Research, Exeter, Devon: Washington Singer Press.

British Medical Association (BMA) (2003) *Housing and Health: Building for the Future*, London: BMA.

Consumers in NHS Research and the Medical Research Council Clinical Trials Unit (2000) *Report of a Seminar: Involving Consumers in Randomized Controlled Trials*, Consumers in NHS Research and the Medical Research Council Clinical Trials Unit (available http://www.invo.org.uk).

Crawford, M.J., Rutter, D., Manley, C., Weaver, T., Bhui, K., Fulop, N. and Tyrer, P. (2002) 'Systematic review of involving patients in the planning and development of health care', *British Medical Journal*, 325: 1263–7.

Department of Health (2001) *A Research and Development Strategy for Public Health*, London: DoH.

Elliott, E., Landes, R., Popay, J. and Edmans, T. (2001) *Regeneration and Health: A Selected Review of Research (Report)*, Leeds: Nuffield Institute for Health, University of Leeds.

Gay, T. (1994) *Barton, Watcombe and Hele (Torquay) Health Gain Initiative*, Report to the Plymouth and Torbay Health Authority.

Hanley, B., Bradburn, J., Gorin, S., Barnes, M., Evans, C., Goodare, H., Kelson, M., Kent, A., Oliver, S. and Wallcraft, J. (2000) *Report of Consumers in NHS Research Support Unit: Involving Consumers in Research and Development in the NHS – Briefing Notes for Researchers*, Eastleigh, Hampshire.

Hanley, B., Truesdale, A., King, A., Elbourne, D. and Chalmers, I. (2001) 'Involving consumers in designing, conducting, and interpreting randomised controlled trials: questionnaire survey', *British Medical Journal*, 322: 519–23.

Molyneux, P. (2003) 'How residents know best', Paper presented at the Conference UnHealthy Housing: Promoting Good Health, University of Warwick.

Somerville, M., Barton, A., Foy, C. and Basham, M. (on behalf of the Torbay Healthy Housing Group) (2001) 'From local concern to randomized trial: the Watcombe Housing Project', presentation at the Society of Social Medicine and the International Epidemiological Association European Group Joint Conference, Oxford.

Somerville, M., Basham, M., Foy, C., Ballinger, G., Gay, T., Shute, P. and Barton, A. (2002) 'From local concern to randomised trial: the Watcombe Housing Project', *Health Expectations*, 5 (2): 127–35.

Stockton, D. and Basham, M. (2002) *Working Together – the Watcombe Housing Project*, London: Consumers in NHS Research Seminar.

University of Bristol (2000) *Housing Management and Sustainable Communities: Video made on behalf of the Institute of Housing*, ISBN nos. Video 1 900396 793, Bristol: Institute of Housing Conference, University of Bristol.

Chapter 11

Helping older people to share the research journey

Mary Leamy

Introduction

Consider the following piece of reflective writing from Clare, one of the older people who undertook research for the Housing Decisions in Old Age (HDOA) study:

> For most of my adult life I had been totally occupied – raising children, always surrounded by young people, I was constantly challenged both mentally and physically. Life was a 'full on' experience and packed with ever changing interests and goals. When you're focused and have aims, time passes very quickly and you are 'too young and too busy to be growing older'! I suppose, on reflection, it was the approaching change in my finances when the truth of my situation began to take on, what seemed to me to be, a sinister perspective. I was used to the word 'pensioner', but all of a sudden, I was approaching the time when society classed me as an 'Old Age Pensioner'. That, and a now deathly quiet and empty house, made me face up to the fact I had reached the time that I always knew would come. Someday! That is when I realized I did not cope with 'negativity' at all well. To simply fill in time was an anathema to me, and as I saw it, very, very negative. It was a very lonely and unsettling time and it lasted for five years, believe it or not!
>
> The mythical 'white knight' comes in many guises. In my case, he wore the cloak of an advertisement from the Department of Continuing Education at Lancaster University. They asked for applications for a course teaching 'The Theory and Practice of Social Research'. The only criterion was that all applicants should be over the age of 60. Bingo! This was the way forward for me if they would accept me as a non-academic. My faith in my abilities, and myself, was instantly reinvigorated when I received the call to tell me I had been accepted. The icing on the cake at that point was when I received a *student* parking pass. 'Old Age Pensioner'? No thanks, not for me, too negative. To me, the word 'student' was non-discriminatory and was synonymous with positive thinking. I was moving forward again!

Clare's writing gives an insight into some of her reasons for being involving in the research by undertaking the course. She writes about her raised hopes and expectations that it might rescue her from having to 'fill in time' and give her a new challenge to focus her energies upon in her retirement. She also sees it as an opportunity to confront ageism and the stereotypical views about what older people can do.

In this chapter, the analogy of a journey is used to try to convey some of the experiences of including older people in the research process. As academic researchers, we knew the overall destination was to have 200 in-depth interviews carried out by older researchers, but have to confess to not always knowing exactly how we were all going to get there. A journey of this sort is, in part, a trip into the unknown and not everything can be anticipated or planned. We knew why we were embarking upon this journey, but it became important to tune into the motivations and needs of the older people whom we had invited to join us.

'The packing': preparing for the journey

It seemed that the initial 'packing' list for the journey kept expanding, and that the more we thought about the implications of each item, the more complicated the whole endeavour became. A selection of the key research planning dilemmas are set out in Table 11.1 on page 122 and then discussed in more detail in the remainder of this chapter.

Validation

The 'certificate in theory and practice of social research for older people', was developed in collaboration with Lancaster University's Department of Continuing Education (DCE), who ran it as their course, handling the marketing, recruitment and administration. Researchers employed from a research grant carried out the course design and teaching. We decided to get the university to validate the course as a way of trying to ensure older people's research contributions are evaluated positively and taken seriously by policy makers. The validation process helped us to think about what we were trying to do and raised key questions like 'Should the course have credits towards a undergraduate degree?' 'What assessments should students complete?' 'What are the entry requirements for the course?' 'What happens if students fail course requirements?' 'It is unusual for students to be paid for completing fieldwork if it is part of the course requirements, so should they be paid?'

We had set up five panels of older people across Britain to advise us on the research plans and strategy. These were the sorts of dilemmas we put to them. To make the course comparable with other DCE courses, it was established that the certificate would be worth 40 credits and taught at first year, undergraduate degree level, over two academic terms. This led to the inclusion of course assessments, which would meet the validation requirements for 40 credits but, more importantly, would be of benefit to students and enable tutors to judge their ability to carry out interviews for the project. After much deliberation, we decided we needed to have some mechanism for only permitting those students who had reached an acceptable standard to conduct interviews. To do this, students were required to pass the first, taught module before being allowed to take the second 'fieldwork' module and carry out the HDOA interviews. Although with sufficient time and effort, it may have been possible to get everyone to the required level of expertise, this is a good example of research and teaching obligations being in conflict. In this case, research considerations took priority and it was made clear to students at the outset that that this was necessary. Out of the Lancaster and London cohorts, only one student failed module one.

Table 11.1 The initial 'to do' list

Research activities	Teaching and research issues	Further implications
Equip older people with the skills to conduct in-depth interviews	What type of course?	Skills based training or education in research methods? University accredited with formal assessment requirements or less formal training?
	How to develop course to teach them?	What do they need to know? How long do they need to learn this? Research staff have to develop teaching skills
	How to market the course?	Who is the target audience? How to recruit enough students to make course viable?
	Other recruitment issues?	What are the selection criteria? Should we use the application forms and/or interviews?
	How to fund the course?	Who pays? Where does the money come from?
Ensure quality of interviews sufficient to fully answer research questions	How to support older people's HDOA fieldwork?	Think of how to give individual feedback, meet regularly to pick up other issues
	Ways of monitoring interview quality?	Should students successfully complete certificate before conducting fieldwork, or should fieldwork be part of the course requirements?
	How to regularly review and revise interview schedule?	Make sure potential or actual difficulties are identified early
	What about theoretical sampling?	Get famililiar with interview transcripts and do preliminary data analysis to be able to spot gaps in data
Complete the target	Sample representativeness	Need to include people living in urban, metropolitan areas not just rural Think about running two courses, one in Lancaster and one in London
	Other sampling issues?	Need to generate interview sample in time for fieldwork stage Extra resources may be needed

Funding

The issue of funding was hotly debated in the older people's panels. The idea of asking people to pay for the privilege of being involved in research seemed at odds with the philosophy of participatory research. A compromise was reached whereby students were asked to make a token contribution to the costs of running the course as a way of getting an initial commitment, but the fees were heavily subsidized from the research grant. Students received payment for each of the interviews they completed as part of second module, so they recouped the course fees and were in profit at the end.

Like other DCE courses, the fees were charged on a variable scale; with all students receiving further discounts because they were of pensionable age and some because they were also in receipt of the state pension. With the benefit of hindsight, we would have increased the payment per interview as the students had to pay income tax on their earnings and complete lengthy tax forms to have this reimbursed (for more on initial preparations, see Leamy and Clough 2001). This issue became contentious and many chose not to bother reclaiming the tax.

In a review of 26 training initiatives for service user involvement in health and social care research, Lockey et al. (2004) found that participants were rarely paid for attending training, but this had led to some participants questioning the fairness of this situation if employed researchers also attended the training.

Marketing and recruitment

As well as advertising the course in the usual way, via the *Continuing Education newspaper*, students were also recruited via the University of the Third Age and Age Concern networks. Writing articles for local newspapers was particularly effective because it reportedly captured people's imagination and led to the recruitment of many individuals who would not normally consider applying for university courses. The courses were open access and the only entry requirement was being aged 60 years or over.

Course development

A detailed report from a teaching perspective is available elsewhere (see Leamy and Clough 2004), but the key areas covered within the course are summarized below.

Demystify research process

- What is social research?
- How do you do social research?
- Why did we design project the way we did?

Understanding the research topic

- Share our knowledge and understanding of topic (read draft literature review, prepare handouts, recommended reading lists).
- Videos of BBC's *When I Get Older* series for group discussions.
- Listen to students' existing understanding and experience of topic.

Skills training component

- How to manage the interview – techniques, styles, anticipating problems, ethics, good 'research etiquette', explaining and answering questions on the project.
- Learn and practise how to use recording equipment.
- Practise using interview schedules flexibly, knowing how and when to prompt for more information.

Supervising interviews

- Ensure interviewers felt well supported.
- Monitor progress of individual interviewers.
- Monitor quality of overall data collected.

Analysis and interpretation

- Learn and practise how to analyse qualitative material.
- Discuss own interpretations.

Learning how to teach

Early on, it became evident that we would need to develop teaching skills. The course had evolved from the original idea of running a short three-day skills training course into something more ambitious, aiming to educate older people about research methods, spread over a longer timescale. This meant familiarizing ourselves with teaching issues like planning course content, sequencing and learning resources, selecting the teaching, learning and assessment methods, thinking about how to provide student support and evaluate the course. Fortunately, the university's certificate in learning and teaching in higher education was available to researchers who were engaged in teaching. Taking this two-year course while planning and delivering the certificate in research methods was arduous and time-consuming, but for a novice teacher, the access to peer and tutor support was invaluable.

Hazards, diversions and roadblocks: a risky journey

Ultimately, from many perspectives, we judged the journey to have been hugely worthwhile. However, there is a danger in forgetting, or perhaps choosing not to remember, the potential hazards, diversions and roadblocks that were faced along the way. While not wishing to put anyone else off this sort of approach, the intention here is to provide an honest account of our experience in taking this route.

Teaching research methods: module one

In university teaching, designing a curriculum with an eye on student retention has become increasingly important, but for us, student dropout took on added dimensions. The student outcomes – whether they were able or motivated to finish the course at all, achieve a satisfactory standard and complete their quota of interviewees – would all have impacted upon the research outcomes. Had the first course in Lancaster failed, either because there were not enough applicants, too many students dropped out, or failed the first module, the whole research strategy would have needed reworking, leading to serious deadline and financial implications. To guard against these scenarios we made strenuous efforts to market the course and deliberately over-recruited student numbers. In Lancaster, of the seventeen students who started the course, three dropped out very early on when they had a better understanding of what it entailed and a further two dropped out at the assessment stage. Of the thirteen students recruited in London, three dropped out at the assessment stage.

Supervising the fieldwork: module two

Safety

Before the interviewers started their fieldwork, it was necessary to put some safety procedures into place. For example, there were issues around liability (interviewers were covered by university insurance), interviewer safety (they were given training and instructions of procedures to follow to ensure their safety) and interviewee safety (interviewers supplied references and completed application form, based on registered charities' policies for recruiting volunteers).

Sampling

While we were explaining the interview sampling strategy to the Lancaster students, we asked them for ideas of how older people in more remote, rural areas could be reached. As a result, they volunteered to put notices up in their villages, adverts in parish newsletters and generally help publicize the project via word-of-mouth. It was an excellent way of building the sample through using 'snowballing' techniques and gave the students an opportunity to develop their role in an unexpected way. It had occurred to us that students could help us generate the sample, but we had been reluctant to ask, thinking it might be perceived as a chore. We knew we were already expecting a considerable commitment from students. They had told us informally that the course was more demanding than they had anticipated – one student had said it was harder than his Open University course. In the end, about 20 per cent of the 189 interviews conducted were developed through student contacts. When the course was repeated in London, we deliberately took advantage of this turn of events by trying even harder to actively recruit students from ethnic minorities, so they could interview within their own communities if they wished.

It was necessary to anticipate and overcome practical organizational issues like synchronizing timing of generation of interview sample with the time students were ready to start the fieldwork stage, and ensuring there was a continuous sample of interviewees throughout the fieldwork stage. Allocating interviewees to interviewers was an important but time-consuming task, which required matching geographical locations and making sure that interviewers without their own transport could get to interviewees' homes using public transport. In London, for example, there were serious delays in identifying the interview sample. Luckily, by this time, the students were sufficiently motivated and committed to the project that they understood the difficulties and were very patient. This was a dangerous time though; having put in the time, effort and funds to run the course for three months, it would have been devastating if they decided not to continue. From their perspective, it was very frustrating to have to wait, hard to maintain the momentum, and difficult having to remember and apply their newly acquired skills when the gaps between interviews became more drawn out.

Support and supervision

The key reason for designing the course in two parts and running it over two academic terms was to enable us to build in sufficient supervision time. Having regular fortnightly supervision sessions served a number of important functions and provided:

- social contact and support from fellow students
- technical guidance on interviewing performance from tutors
- time for in-depth discussion and exchanging ideas on research topic
- an opportunity to monitor quality of interviews by checking the data obtained was relevant to the research aims
- the chance to discuss and deal with fieldwork issues as they arose.

Students were given the choice of individual or group supervision sessions. They opted for group sessions, even though this meant allowing others to read their transcripts and receiving their individual interview feedback in public. Splitting each cohort into two kept the supervision groups to a manageable size. Giving feedback required considerable tact and skill, but from looking at the transcripts together, students were usually able to spot places to improve their interviewing technique and style for themselves. Usually the feedback was a collection of suggestions on how the interview could have been developed by spotting opportunities to ask important follow-up questions. This enabled supervision sessions to quickly move from being an exercise in improving interview technique to learning how to understand and explore the topic more deeply.

It is our belief that getting this level of supervision on research methods courses is unusual. Indeed, many academic researchers do not receive such detailed feedback on their individual interviews. At one stage, we began to wonder whether we were being harder on the students than we would be on ourselves. The process was extremely time-consuming, with a short turn-around between receiving interview tapes, handing them to a professional transcriber and tutors getting the transcripts back to read and prepare feedback for the next supervision session. The students were desperate for feedback, wanting our verdict on whether their interviews had been useful. They told us they found the experience valuable, and the improvements in the quality of the interviews definitely made it worth the effort. At the same time, it also provided the first opportunity for us to read, become familiar with each interviewee's story, and begin theorizing and developing ideas from what had been said.

Fortnightly group sessions were important in picking up and managing fieldwork issues as they arose. For instance, some of the interviewers felt a profound sense of responsibility towards their interviewees, occasionally being drawn into situations where they felt over-extended, helpless, emotionally exhausted and unsure how to extract themselves from their involvement. Having an opportunity to discuss the boundaries and nature of the researcher–interviewee relationship was very important. For the research project, one of the many advantages of working with a charity like Counsel and Care was the ready access to sources of help like information leaflets, telephone help lines and specialist advice workers. Having this support in place went some way to enabling interviewers to feel more comfortable dealing with these types of issues.

Fellow travellers

Part of trying to understand how to successfully involve those who would normally be 'research subjects' in the research process is about understanding what makes a good travelling companion. How can this relationship become established, then developed and maintained?

Direction and purpose

We believe the distinctiveness of the approach described here lies in the integration and co-dependence of research and teaching practice. We know of a few recent or ongoing examples of running courses to equip older people to carry out research, but they required participants to initiate their own research projects. By merging research and teaching in an unusual way, students were given the opportunity to engage in a real-life, ongoing social research project that served to unite them in a common venture that had credibility, a clear set of aims, objectives, timetable and outcomes. The research topic, while not originally selected by them, was recognized as being pertinent to their own lives, and students were clearly motivated to complete the course and the research tasks to the best of their ability.

Hopes and fears

At the outset, we had to try to find a way of sharing our research vision, which included our hopes and fears of what may lie ahead. To be able to do this in a way that would make sense, we recognized that we also needed to demystify the research process and share our knowledge of research theory, process, methods, and issues with students. It was not a matter of simply getting them to do the legwork for us and conduct interviews without understanding the bigger picture.

To try to appreciate where the students were coming from, very early on, we asked them to explain to us their motivations for doing the course and reveal their hopes and fears about completing it. This was a revealing and useful way for us to learn about and respond to their concerns and adapt the approach accordingly. We tried to find ways to continually check with the students how they were feeling about the course and the research – asking them informally, but also getting them to write about it as part of their assessed work. Part of the task for us centred on responding to the students' needs and managing their expectations.

The expectations–reality gap

Although we broadly knew where we were going and how to get there, some of the details of how to achieve this had to be worked out as we went along. It clearly is not possible to plan and anticipate everything beforehand. With hindsight, we freely admit we underestimated the demands on the students and ourselves. It was hard to tell the Lancaster students what to expect because we were also new to this way of working and did not really know what to expect either. We were more prepared when we reran the certificate in London. The course was tough and introduced many new ideas and skills in a relatively short space of time. Sharing the research journey with older people means also sharing the messiness, dead-ends and uncertainty that always accompany the research process, but which researchers rarely admit to. The fact that so many students stuck with us and completed the course successfully, despite such demands, provides compelling evidence of their single-minded determination and impressive perseverance.

Roles and communication

We learnt how 'sharing the messiness' of the research process comes with its own problems and tensions. In establishing roles and relationships, we needed to convince students that we were credible researchers so that they would have confidence in what we were doing. This 'expert' role needed to be balanced with an 'empowering' or 'facilitative' role where we created an atmosphere in which students felt able to challenge us and propose alternative ways of doing things. A key benefit of involving older people in research is their ability to challenge invalid assumptions made by younger researchers. This benefit is lost if older people do not feel confident enough to question the authority of academic researchers.

The mismatch of professional and service user communication styles, and the associated problems for working together, have been identified before. Church (1995) has argued that these need to be overcome for professional–user collaboration to become more effective. From a teaching perspective, rather than choosing to ban the use of academic language entirely, we tried to minimize it and, where its use was unavoidable, explain each term at the time, handing out glossaries of research terminology as a memory aid.

Making mistakes

> It's not just a course with you teaching research methods, but everybody learning together.
>
> (London research student)

The style we stumbled on within the course can perhaps best be described as 'learning together'. Certainly, everyone had a lot to learn quickly and usually this was from 'learning by doing'. Being prepared to be tolerant of one another's mistakes, and allowing sufficient time and space to learn from them, is clearly part of this process. The experiences of buying and operating the tape recorders serves as a good case in point. We realized, too late, that older people had not been involved in the selection of the tape-recording equipment. Although the model that was selected appeared to be one of the most suitable on the market for our recording purposes, it was not ideal for use by older people. The buttons were small and awkward to use and the lettering that marked recording level settings was too small to read. We had also underestimated how uncomfortable and anxious students would initially be about their ability to operate the tape recorders. In practice, the recording equipment, both recorders and tapes, were sometimes unreliable, adding to the difficulties. Coupled with the occasional mistakes made by students, some interviews were not recorded at all or were of poor sound quality, and consequently difficult or impossible to transcribe. Of course, most researchers, if they were honest, could probably tell a few 'horror' stories of their own around using recording equipment. Through this process of trial and error, we began to learn that when we did not know what to do, asking ourselves 'Is this in the spirit of involvement?' often helped.

Saying goodbyes and starting new journeys

While the work associated with the Housing Decisions in Old Age study is ending, it has not meant ending the working relationships with former students. At the time of writing, around ten people who completed the certificate in social research methods in the North West have set themselves up as a co-operative called Older People Researching Social Issues (OPRSI) and are now offering their services as qualified, experienced social interviewers. OPRSI have just completed a one-year project, funded by the Joseph Rowntree Foundation, called 'Older People as Researchers: Potential, Practicalities and Pitfalls', continuing their collaboration with two members of the HDOA research team – Roger Clough (research director) and Les Bright (former deputy chief executive, Counsel and Care). During this time, with Les and Roger's help and contacts, they have also undertaken smaller research contracts with local charities and authorities, and have been asked to participate in training activities and writing research proposals.

In another exciting development, OPRSI are taking part in a larger two-year, Department of Health funded project, on 'User–professional relationships in social and health care' that is being managed by Glasgow University. The central research task will be conducting 120/360 interviews with NHS service users about the effectiveness of user–professional partnerships and provide an excellent opportunity to join new research networks of academic and user researchers. This is crucial if OPRSI are to be able to become more established, better resourced and less reliant upon a handful of key individuals for their survival. As an interim step, funds to pay for my own services to provide a part-time, local supportive/ facilitative role has been included in the research proposal, providing a welcome opportunity to re-establish contact with OPRSI.

Parting thoughts

Changing worlds, changing titles

Much writing on participation, indeed the title of this book, relates to people who are service users. It is worth noting that older people who become involved in research may or may not be users of social and health care services, though they could be described as potential service users. To get around this, others have coined the term 'lay researchers'. During the duration of the research, we jointly struggled to find an suitable title that would do justice to them and the nature of their involvement: 'students'; 'team members'; 'older interviewers'; 'user researchers'; 'novice researchers'? While some were better than others, none of these were quite right. For instance, the original term 'older interviewers', although appropriate at the outset, soon became too restrictive in terms of activity and did not fully portray the complexities of our relationship. On reflection, it more closely resembled a relationship between a research supervisor and postgraduate research student, which starts out with an academic expert and inexperienced student but, over a number of years, moves towards one in which students develop their own expertise and confidence to challenge their supervisors. While the title 'student' was most popular, of course on successful completion of the certificate, it no longer applied. For the time being, the title 'older researcher' has stuck, perhaps because it best captures what is distinctive about what they can offer over 'academic researchers'.

The older researchers were in a similar position to most research associates who are recruited by the research grant holders only after the proposal has been developed and funded. Arguably, their situation is comparable to that of some research associates who register for a postgraduate degree while conducting the funded research, requiring an element of 'learning on the job'. There is potential not only for conflict between the demands of the degree and the requirements of employers but also for research associates to enhance their commitment and their personal stake in the research outcome. They join the research team when much preparatory work and thinking has been done and they need to familiarize themselves with the project before they can contribute effectively.

Was it really worth it?

For everyone, the ultimate test of 'success' was always whether the research interview data could be used to develop theories and understanding of older people's housing decisions. We recently concluded that it could:

> Sharing the research journey with older people who would traditionally only be invited to take on the roles of interviewee or questionnaire respondent, has been immensely rewarding and satisfying for us personally, as well as being beneficial for the research. It is hard to capture succinctly the effect collaborating in this way has had. Perhaps it is best to let the quality of the interviews drawn upon in this book speak for themselves.
>
> (Clough et al. 2004:)

Acknowledgements

In addition to Mary Leamy, the academic team included Roger Clough (research director), Vince Miller (research associate, Lancaster University), Les Bright (deputy chief executive) and Liz Brooks (project officer, Council and Care).

References

Church, K. (1995) *Forbidden Narratives: Critical Autobiography as Social Science*, New York and London: Gordon and Breach.

Clough, R., Leamy, M., Miller, V. with Bright, L. (2004) *Housing Decisions in Later Life*, Basingstoke: Palgrave Macmillan.

Leamy, M. and Clough, R. (2001) 'Older people as researchers: their role in a research project', *Education and Ageing*, 16 (3): 279–87.

Leamy, M. and Clough, R. (2005) *Depending on Each Other: Teaching, Researching and Older People's Perspectives on Doing Research Together*, York: Joseph Rowntree Foundation.

Lockey, R., Sitzia, J., Gillingham, T., Millyard, J., Miller, C., Ahmed, S., Beales, A., Bennet, C., Parfoot, S., Sigrist, G. and Sigrist, J. (2004) *Training for Service User Involvement in Health and Social Care Research: A Study of Training Provision and Participants' Experiences* (The TRUE project), Worthing, Sussex: Worthing and Southlands Hospitals NHS Trust.

Chapter 12

Really making it happen in Wiltshire

The experience of service users evaluating social care

Clare Evans and Ray Jones

Introduction

This chapter grows out of learning from our shared agenda and working together over ten years (since 1992) in promoting user involvement in social care to improve the quality of social care services. Ray Jones has been the director of Social Services in Wiltshire since 1992, a chiefly rural local authority and Clare Evans is the founder, former director and now president of Wiltshire and Swindon Users Network, a user controlled organization formed in 1991 and registered as a limited co-operative company in 1993. From this shared experience, we shall describe the growing user led context in which examples of users involved in research and evaluation of services developed. These examples range from ongoing informal research through regular focus groups, through involvement in particular parts of research to carrying out formal user controlled research and evaluation.

Background context

Service users formed Wiltshire and Swindon Users Network (WSUN) in response to the new opportunities for user involvement in community care enshrined in the legislation of the Community Care NHS Act 1991. Alongside the development of a separate carers' network, community development techniques were used to contact individual users and groups of users to meet together at regular meetings. These meetings enabled users to gain information about aspects of community care implementation such as care management, share experiences, support each other and feel safe to speak out together – in short, to empower themselves. Over twelve years later in 2003, user members continued to identify these aspects as valuable WSUN activities in formal research they conducted as part of a partnership review with funders (Evans and Evans 2004). In 1991, the users involved were also proactive in lobbying to be involved in various aspects of social care planning and delivery such as workshops to design care management processes and documentation and care management training of health and social service staff. For example, the views of different stakeholders and the good practice required from the experience of users as participants in staff training is documented by Evans and Hughes (1993).

While service users in Wiltshire were organizing and developing their own organization in response to needs they identified, there was a parallel development within the Disabled People's Movement. This involved the self-organization of disabled people, chiefly with physical and sensory impairments, into local campaigning groups based on the social model of disability identifying the social barriers to their full participation as citizens in society. In Wiltshire, Social Services senior management's commitment to invite users to design a third party scheme to enable users to purchase their own care prior to legislation to legalize Direct Payments, led to WSUN members becoming more politicized. They were exposed to concepts of independent living based on the Social Model of Disability as they networked with other disabled people developing similar schemes in their own localities.

However, WSUN had several distinctive features, which enabled it to be more focused and effective at developing user involvement and lobbying for change in social care than traditional models of local groups of disabled people. It actively encourages membership from all user perspectives and sought to stress members' common experience of oppression as long-term users while providing space for them to meet with others in their own care groups to give their views on services relevant to their needs. WSUN developed as a countywide network of service users committed to outreach to those marginalized users, stressing the value of each user's experience and accountability rather than 'a representation of' other users' views. Moreover, WSUN's mission statement specified its purpose as relating to the empowerment of service users and promoting change within social care. While based on the principles of disability equality and the social model, the focus of activity was primarily on health and social care, although at times it was relevant to lobby other services in line with a commitment to and aspirations to the same quality of life as other citizens.

Meanwhile, developments back in Social Services as 'Community Care' was implemented emphasized that the Community Care changes were about increasing participation and choice for service users. Within the 'care management' process, the focus was to be on discussion with service users about their views of the difficulties they might be experiencing, the need for assistance they had and how this assistance might best be provided, albeit within the rationing requirements resulting from cash limited budgets and eligibility criteria of the local authority.

The use of the Community Care specific transitional grant from the Department of Health created an initially uncommitted cash budget that could be used flexibly to meet the needs and wishes of service users, and with the emphasis throughout on providing more assistance to enable service users to live independently in their own homes and their own communities. Those service users who needed and agreed to move into residential care were given a choice (the national 'choice directive') of at least three residential homes that, if necessary, social services would assist them to visit.

In developing more flexible, creative and responsive local services for service users, 'link workers' were employed across Wiltshire. They were based within primary care settings, such as GP practices and local health centres. Most of their time was to be spent on care management and building links between GPs, district nurses and the area social services offices, but 25 per cent of their time was to be spent on developing local services to respond to what was identified locally as 'unmet need'.

Local service development, included, for example, getting a local supermarket to do home deliveries or a village pub to prepare meals for older people, where the old people might meet together to have their meal in the pub or the meals might be delivered by local volunteers. Throughout, service users were involved in service planning and development, and in training care managers to make them more aware of the experience, and indeed expertise, of service users.

By 1995, WSUN calculated their user members were involved in over 60 different ways within Social and Health Services. As professional workers became more confident about their new role and processes within Community Care, and a more user led culture developed within Social Services, attention locally turned to definitions of quality and collecting service users' views as a way of measuring effectiveness of services. Within this climate, it was a natural development for service users to become involved in research on evaluating services and identifying gaps in service provision.

What was of particular significance was how service users 'riddled' the planning and commissioning systems which were developed across Wiltshire. This included service users being involved in all planning groups, which became a requirement and tradition throughout Wiltshire for children and families services as well as adult-focused Community Care services. Service users were involved from the beginning in setting agendas, rather than being invited towards the end of the process to comment on consultative documents, in the drawing up of tender specifications and in evaluating and selecting service providers through the commissioning and contracting processes. Service users also took the lead in planning, commissioning and reviewing services themselves, such as advocacy services.

One gain from the planning and commissioning processes was that service users were able to influence the development of health and housing services as well as social care. For example, a NHS respite care service for disabled people provided in an ageing local hospital that was to close was replaced by an independent sector company, which was commissioned to provide a purpose-built respite care residential home. Service users were involved in designing the specification for the new service, in selecting the provider and subsequently in monitoring and reviewing the service. Service users were also central to, and involved throughout, the planning, commissioning and tendering of a housing development where disabled people now live independently receiving assistance either from a care agency who were selected to provide an on-site service or through separately and individually recruited personal assistants.

Informal research from user focus groups

An important part of WSUN's operating objectives was to have local user only focus groups for all care groups at regular intervals across the county. One purpose of these was to provide Social Services with users' views of their services and the gaps in provision. These groups were facilitated by a user development worker, employed by WSUN to provide a safe environment with no fear of repercussions. The worker collected the views collectively and informed WSUN's policy's co-ordinator and the local statutory planning officers. Users had their travel costs paid to attend meetings. These could be considerable in a rural county where taxis could be a necessity. Other considerations to make the focus groups effective were planning meetings at accessible venues, at convenient times, providing refreshments and running the meeting in a form accessible to all participants.

This was at times a most effective way to monitor services and gaps in provision. For example, a theme emerging from focus groups across the county was the widespread unmet need identified by older people to have toenails regularly trimmed. Health service chiropodists were able to cater only for those with more complex foot problems, and home care staff were advised by managers not to perform this task for health and safety and 'litigation' reasons. Lobbying on this matter centrally led to a response by senior managers to address the issue. Some years later, it was possible for this service to be offered by home carers after training from chiropodists.

What made the difference here, in getting a proposal from service users finally enacted, was perseverance by service users. Over time, there was increasing understanding of the experience of service users (e.g. how poor foot care made it difficult and painful for service users to remain as independent as they wanted). There was increasing recognition that current arrangements were not efficient and easily accessible (e.g. a fully professionally trained foot care specialist is not needed for every foot care task, and that waiting times and centralized locations for chiropodists created difficulties for service users who were having difficulty walking anyway). There was also increasing confidence that properly trained and supervised home carers (who were already undertaking many more personal care tasks) could within their expanded role undertake some foot care (such as filing nails).

User research in partnership

Our organizations' shared agenda to improve services led to several opportunities for joint monitoring of new initiatives piloted to improve and integrate service delivery between Health and Social Services. In a pilot project sponsored by the King's Fund, Wiltshire was one of six sites exploring the joint commissioning of services (Poxton 1996; Challis and Pearson 1996). Older service users active in WSUN sat on the pilot steering group to review progress regularly in this action research and led new initiatives to meet gaps in services such as on community based 'handihelp' schemes. They also encouraged other older people to give their views by leading focus groups of older people receiving services in the pilot geographical area. An important principle expounded by WSUN, which the pilot steering group signed up to, was user only meetings with older people acting as role models leading them to underpin the planning of services with a wide range of users' views.

In another such initiative, Social Services wanted independent research into older users' views of their experiences of transfer after hospital discharge. Because the relevant users were likely to lack mobility and still be recuperating, it was decided that telephone interviews by trained and experienced service users using semistructured questionnaires was the most appropriate way of collecting data. In this research, it was recognized that peers with similar previous experiences would be empathetic and encourage a more open response from interviewees than others!

WSUN were also involved in the establishment of the University of Bath/Wiltshire Social Services Research and Development Partnership. The University of Bath partnership had been established by Wiltshire County Council's Social Services Department in 1997 as a means of independently researching and evaluating major policy and practice developments within Wiltshire. As part of Social Services commitments to involve users as stakeholders in all initiatives, WSUN were invited to nominate a user to be on the recruitment panel of the partnership director. Through their influence in the selection process, it was possible to ensure the selected candidate would build user involvement into future research proposals developed in the partnership. There were further opportunities for users to contribute to the design of research and scoping exercises for research proposals.

Sometimes it has been appropriate to employ a disabled person as a professional researcher. In addition to having the skills of a professional researcher, it was felt the disabled person would have empathetic skills that would reach out to particularly marginalized users. Thus, a disabled researcher was used to contact and interview young disabled people not linked with any formal groupings and services to identify their aspirations and requirements of services. A large national voluntary organization employed a disabled researcher through the partnership to interview disabled people living in large traditional residential homes about alternative service provision. The problem of gaining the views of disabled people, who have internalized oppression and therefore low aspirations, is well known. A disabled interviewer provides an alternative role model and is able to focus with ease on particular aspects of choice and control, which enables the interviewee to realize the possibility of alternative provision (Carmichael and Brown 2000).

Best Value reviews

The increased emphasis on monitoring the quality of public services led to legislation requiring local authorities to introduce a system of 'Best Value reviews' of service in 1999. This provided a formal framework within which service users could participate in reviewing the services they used. The Best Value review process in Wiltshire County Council included not only, as nationally, the 'four Cs' of consultation, challenge, comparison and competition, but also in Wiltshire the 'C' of collaboration, especially with service users as a part of the Best Value review process to check that services were appropriate and provided value for money.

While service users were routinely asked their views in consultation as part of reviews as required legally, Social Services were also committed to involve users in a more actively participant way from the start, in line with good practice in user involvement generally. Thus, people with learning difficulties were invited to be part of the Best Value board in the review of their services and contributed to the design of methods to collect service users' views of existing services, and continued to participate fully in the partnership board established to implement the design of new services.

User controlled research

At certain times, service users through WSUN chose to conduct their own research enabling them to have control of the whole research process. Barnes and Mercer (1997) describe emancipatory research as having control over the social means of production from the commissioning of research through to its dissemination. From the three pieces of user controlled research published by WSUN, it is possible to note both similarities and differences to other kinds of research.

In its survey of members referred to above (Evans and Evans 2004), WSUN was given the task of designing and carrying out the research to be used by the partnership review as part of evidence to explore the effectiveness of publicly funded work by

WSUN for both service users and Social Services. Elected service users on the management committee designed the survey questions, which were informally consulted on with other service users. Their understanding of the aims of the organization led to questions about WSUN's activities, the accessibility of its information and aspirations of its members for a campaigning agenda based on the social model of disability. While professional researchers might consider the lack of questions about respondents' age, gender, race and impairment as evidence of gender, age, race and disability blindness, it can also be interpreted as demonstrating WSUN's commitment to the lack of importance of these differences in the face of external oppression or just lack of experience in drawing up questionnaires.

The survey was conducted by post and had a response rate of 25 per cent. A user member with experience in market research collated the replies and another analysed the results to present back to the Partnership Review Board. The survey results provided insight into the role WSUN played in preparing and supporting users in the user involvement services provided to statutory authorities. It showed the role that peer support, information provision and collective advocacy played in empowering service users through their own organization.

In earlier research in 1995, WSUN were assisted by an experienced professional researcher acting as an ally as user members conducted research from commissioning to dissemination into the Support Service of Wiltshire Independent Living Fund, which provided support to disabled people purchasing their own care (Collaboratively Wiltshire Users Network 1996). A group of service users interested in the research met regularly to design the different stages of the research. It was funded with £18,000 from Social Services to promote independent living. Four disabled people collected the data by interviewing twenty randomly selected recipients of the Wilts Support Service. Training in interview techniques, and a semistructured interview schedule, were provided to support the inexperienced interviewers. The most difficult research task for users to carry out was the analysis of the interview responses using a corporate method. The professional researcher designed a chart of themes against which the results could be collated and analysed. Although the research was published, and lessons drawn out about user controlled research methodology, the research was not used by the service users to influence policy (Evans and Fisher 1999).

Later research commissioned by WSUN and funded by the Joseph Rowntree Foundation sought to demonstrate service users' ability to carry out Best Value reviews of services and to influence the local authority policy on Direct Payments (Evans and Carmichael 2002). WSUN members were assisted by professional allies in the Joseph Rowntree Foundation and the Bath University Wiltshire Partnership to prepare the research brief to submit for funding. Again, the research design was developed by an interested group of disabled people of both sexes with a range of ages and impairments. But, in this research a disabled professional researcher committed to emancipatory research facilitated the user group and carried out the research by methods identified by them.

In 2000, as the pattern of Best Value reviews was developing, senior managers within the local authority were able to accommodate the philosophy of user control within the Best Value structures. The research directors from WSUN and the Bath Partnership became the Best Value project managers, and the Best Value Project

Board included service users and was advisory rather than managerial. The external challenger was a disabled person managing a direct payments scheme in a neighbouring local authority area. In their turn, the WSUN research group kept to the Best Value review timescales and report deadlines required by the local authority.

The user research group met monthly to design a variety of research methods to collect evidence for the review. They designed a survey to circulate to all direct payments users and chose themselves to interview care managers about their knowledge and experience of direct payments. Some members of the group kept diaries of their day-to-day experience of using direct payments and others designed a questionnaire to collect data from Direct Payment Support Service schemes in other areas to compare with the Wiltshire one. In this project, the group wanted to use the research to influence the direct payments scheme locally and the Best Value review report was a vehicle to achieve this. To maintain influence over the ensuing action plan the local authority would develop in response to the report recommendations, they recommended the setting up of an ongoing user monitoring group. The research findings showed the need for more training on direct payments for care managers, for a central office management of direct payments and for changes in the financial systems and in regulations related to the use of direct payments for equipment purchase. The users' aim to influence local policy in carrying out the research dictated the priorities of dissemination identified by the user research group. They arranged a local launch inviting Social Services professions and direct payments users, at which they presented their findings and recommendations. A national launch was arranged later that sought to disseminate the learning about user involvement in Best Value reviews to academics and professionals.

A Best Value review shaped, directed and undertaken by service users had, from the perspective of the county council, the benefits of being truly independent and informed throughout by the experience and expertise of service users. This made it more likely that the outcome of the review would be relevant and meaningful to service users, focusing on their experience and what was most important to them.

It was, however, also a risk for the county council. No longer would it be possible for the county council to put its spin on the review findings and how these were presented. The questions asked within the review would also primarily be the questions that were most important for service users, which could be uncomfortable and particularly challenging for the council. There was also the risk that the Best Value review undertaken by service users would not meet the review criteria set by the Audit Commission and against which the council would be assessed and rated as it was still held accountable for the application of the Audit Commission's review process.

The outcome of the review has had significant positive impact on direct payment processes in Wiltshire. An independent monitoring report (Carmichael 2004), undertaken by a researcher who is herself a disabled person, shows improvement in payment reliability, support, and information for people considering or using direct payments.

An important good practice principle of user involvement in research is the recognition of the value of users' expertise by the payment of a fee for their contribution. In Wiltshire, we were able to build on the learning from our more general user involvement. From the start, statutory funders recognized that part of WSUN's funding would be used to pay service users an hourly fee for their participation in staff training days and other work with professionals. In relation to research, we extended the principle so that for tasks requiring particular expertise and training, such as interviewing, a higher rate of fee was paid. The good practice guidelines for Wiltshire contributed to the paper developed by INVOLVE (formerly Consumers in NHS Research) giving guidance on this matter to display on their web page to assist other researchers.

Conclusion

So, over a period of more than ten years, service users in Wiltshire, through the establishment of their own independent user controlled organization, have had significant impacts on policy and practice development. One way users have had impact has been through service users independently commissioning, and independently undertaking, research on the experience of service users and on the services they receive. Service users themselves have developed expertise in research, in seeking independent funding, shaping methodology, and acting as interviewers, data analysts and report writers. The service users have developed alliances with other experienced non-disabled researchers to draw on their experience and expertise, but with the service users remaining in charge and in control. For the local authority, and other service providers (including housing, health, library services and environmental planning), the research undertaken by service users has been influential in reshaping policy and practice.

It has not always been comfortable, sometimes it has been particularly challenging, but it has been a win-win for all involved.

References

Barnes, C. and Mercer, G. (1997) 'Breaking the mould? An introduction to doing disability research', in C. Barnes and G. Mercer (eds) *Doing Disability Research*, Leeds: Disability Press.

Carmichael, A. (2004) *Direct Payments Monitoring Review: Survey Findings*, Trowbridge: Wiltshire County Council.

Carmichael, A. and Brown, L. (2000) *Exploring the Accommodation and Support Needs of Disabled People*, Bath: University of Bath and Associates, for the Leonard Cheshire Organisation.

Challis, L. and Pearson, J. (1996) *Getting in Step: A Guide to Practice-based Joint Commissioning*, Bath: University of Bath.

Collaboratively Wiltshire Users Network (1996) *I am in Control – User-controlled Research into Wiltshire Independent Living Fund*, Devizes: Wiltshire and Swindon Users Network.

Evans, C. and Carmichael A. (2002) *Users' Best Value: A Guide to Good Practice in User Involvement in Best Value Reviews*, York: Joseph Rowntree Foundation.

Evans, C. and Evans, R. (2004) 'What users have to say about their own organisations: a local user-controlled study', *Journal of Integrated Care*, 12 (3): 38–46.

Evans, C. and Fisher, M. (1999) 'Collaborative evaluation with service users: moving towards user-controlled research', in I. Shaw and J. Lishman (eds) *Evaluation and Social Work Practice*, London: Sage.

Evans, C. and Hughes, M. (1993) *Tall Oaks from Little Acorns*, Trombridge: Wiltshire Social Services and Wiltshire Users' Network.

Poxton, R. (1996) *Joint Approaches for a Better Old Age*, London: King's Fund.

Chapter 13

Research with children who use NHS services

Sharing the experience

Tina Moules

Introduction

Recognition of the importance of acknowledging the participation rights of young people is now evident throughout current government thinking. The Department of Health (2001), in its introduction to the Children's Taskforce, acknowledges the role young people can play and commits itself to 'ensuring that the voice of the child is heard and correctly acted upon'. Young people's participation underpins the development of the Children's National Service Framework and plays a major role in the Quality Protects programme. In November 2000, the UK government launched the Children and Young People's Unit (CYPU). This cross-departmental unit stresses that central to its work is a 'commitment to engage with children and young people themselves, learning from what works and from each other; to develop services that are better designed and delivered to meet young people's needs' (CYPU 2000: 1). This increased commitment to listen to the views of young people has emerged as a result of a general explosion of interest in them and in their lives, fuelled by the government's need to comply with the articles of the United Nations Convention on the Rights of the Child (UNCRC) 1989 and the Children Act 1989.

Although the commitment is evident on paper, the reality is somewhat different. A survey by Lightfoot and Sloper (2001) noted an apparent growing interest among NHS organizations in involving young people in service development. The survey, of health authorities and NHS Trusts in England, revealed a limited, but growing, range of initiatives involving young people with chronic health problems in decisions about service development. They found that, though all the initiatives included consultation with young people, the majority of initiatives were characterized by limited involvement and in only eleven cases were young people actually involved in the process of decision making. Hennessy (1999) reviewed the literature for evidence of young people's involvement in service evaluation. In the main, though many studies addressed the topic of client satisfaction with paediatric services, most treated parents as the sole client. A limited number of methods for eliciting the views of young people were identified but all used quantitative methods to gather data including postal questionnaires and structured interviews.

Guidelines for involving young people in research and decision making processes are numerous (Save the Children 2002; CYPU 2001; National Children's Bureau (NCB) 2002; Warrell 2000; Kirby 1999; Cohen and Emmanuel 1998; Morris 1998; National Early Years Network (NEYN) 1996). They offer good advice, reasoned principles and examples of methods to use. While this is clearly a step in the right direction, putting policy into practice can be difficult, time-consuming and fraught with constraints. This chapter analyses some of these issues against the backdrop of participatory research with young people who were users of inpatient services. The process of recruiting young people to the project is explored and the degree to which participation can be achieved is debated. In evaluating the participatory process, the role of young people and the researcher at different stages in the project is examined. Finally some feedback from the young people themselves highlights the importance of evaluating the effectiveness of participation. Sharing my experiences will not provide all the answers to what in many cases are complex questions. Instead, the aim is to stimulate further debate and exploration of the issues and, in doing so lead to the development of better research with young people. (In this chapter, the term young people is used to denote both children and young people.)

The research project in brief

The initial aim of the project was to explore if and how young people could be involved in clinical audit. Clinical audit has become a routine part of health service delivery since it was introduced in the 1980s. Although it is a requirement that users of NHS services should influence all stages of the audit process (DoH 1994, 1997; NHS Executive 1996), evidence of the involvement of service users, especially young people, in the audit process has been limited (Kelson 1995, 1997). For this project, nine young people (aged 12–15), all of whom had been users of inpatient services, were recruited initially and took part in individual interviews. Six of these young people decided to continue with the project and joined the participatory phase where they became co-researchers with me. At this stage the young people decided to find out what other young people thought about being involved in monitoring quality. They devised a data collection tool with my help and participated in collecting the data from young people in a local primary school. They then participated in analysing the data and disseminating the findings.

Recruiting young people to research projects

Several factors can affect the ease with which young people are accessed and recruited to participate as users in NHS research. The impact of these factors will depend on the nature of the research topic and the context in which the research is being carried out, but they are likely to be experienced to some degree by all those conducting research with young people. I particularly wanted to recruit young people whose experiences were relevant to the research project (Morris 1998), those who had experience of hospital admissions. A step-by-step approach was taken to gain support from relevant paediatric consultants, ethical approval from two local research ethics committees and agreement for the project from research and development offices. The next step was to contact parents/carers and young people to give them details about the project and invite them to participate. To do this, it was first necessary to comply with the requirements of the Data Protection Act 1998.

The first principle of the Data Protection Act 1998 (Schedule 1 Part 1) clearly states that 'Personal data shall be processed fairly and lawfully and, in particular, shall not be processed unless at least one of the conditions in Schedule 2 (www.hmso.gov.uk/ acts/acts1998/80029—n.htm#sch2) is met'. Schedule 2 lists six conditions, five of which were not met in my project (accessing data was not necessary for performance of a contract, compliance with legal obligations, to protect the data subject, for the purposes of pursuing legitimate interests (treatment) or for the administration of justice). Therefore, the sixth condition *had* to be met – the data subject must 'give their consent to processing'. Strobl et al. (2000) suggest that there are difficulties in interpreting the Act and also to some extent the duty of confidentiality, leading to confusion and a lack of clear policy guidance. They used a case study approach to examine some of the confusion. The question of whether explicit consent was needed from patients to allow the researcher to access medical records was referred to the five NHS Trusts involved. Decisions varied considerably and also involved complex internal discussions such that decisions were delayed up to five months. In my case, my position as a non-NHS employee carrying out non-contracted research meant that I did not have the legal right to access young people's records other than in my capacity as lecturer when carrying out teaching with student nurses. The decisions taken by the Trusts involved in my project meant that consultants had to gain permission from the parents/carers of potential recruits for me to have their contact details. With a total of more than fourteen possible consultants, this process proved to be time-consuming and complex, necessitating a reliance on other people, in particular a number of very busy consultants, and in the end was unproductive. This experience raises one of the main reasons why researchers find it difficult to gain access to young people as they can normally do so only with the co-operation of a number of different 'gatekeepers'.

Gatekeepers are defined by Hek et al. (1996) as those people who attempt to safeguard the interests of others. Any adult with responsibility for a young person's well-being (parent/carer or professional) may act as a gatekeeper. Although gatekeepers can play a vital role in safeguarding young people with regard to research, they can also act to exert power over young people to prevent their voices being heard. In either case, this places the researcher at the end of a long chain of negotiation, as I experienced. Within NHS Trusts, consultants act as the second line of gatekeepers (the first line being local research ethics committees) from whom consent for research with young people is required. Of the fourteen consultants I contacted, only two (both paediatricians) were supportive. They acknowledged the value of the study and gave a firm commitment to it. Unfortunately their communications with parents failed to elicit any further interest. The remaining twelve consultants (none of whom were paediatricians) declined either to respond or to do so positively and, in some cases, simply denied me access to their patients. In effect, this disempowered parents and young people by preventing them from reaching their own decision. Failure to access young people via the Trusts made me rethink my approach and turn to other professional gatekeepers in the hope of successfully recruiting to the project. I contacted the head teachers of two local schools (one primary and one secondary) who were both supportive and co-operative, contacting parents/carers on my behalf.

Researchers will also normally need to gain co-operation from parents or those in loco parentis, and this group of people constitutes the next line of gatekeepers. In my study, most parents who were asked to consider giving consent for their child to participate did not respond. In all cases where a letter was sent directly to the parents, only two responded declaring an interest in the project. After reading the information sheets, however, both failed to respond positively. None of the parents from the primary school (where children were aged 5–11 years) responded. The only positive responses were from parents of ten young people who had indicated their interest to the second head teacher, who had discussed the project with a number of young people (aged 12–16 years) he knew had been inpatients before sending a letter home introducing me. All these parents received information packs, sent as an enclosure in a letter to the children. On meeting with them, it was evident that the communication between them and their children was open and, as Eiser (1993) observed, in this situation, parents rarely have reservations about giving consent for their children to be involved in research. In only one case did the parent as gatekeeper deny me access to his child. This was not explicit denial but implicit, communicated by non-verbal means on the doorstep of their house. I had arranged an interview time with the young person and his mother. On arrival, my knock was answered by his father, who just said 'They are out' without any further clarification. His manner was brusque and he did not offer to prolong the conversation.

My experience can lead us to question some of the factors at play in the decisions made by professional and non-professional gatekeepers (Figure 13.1).

Do all communications necessarily reach the right person? What makes professionals and parents obstruct the involvement of young people in research? Why don't parents respond to letters? Do they discuss the decision with their children and, if not, why not? What factors are more likely to result in positive support from gatekeepers? We could usefully begin to find answers to these questions by considering how adult-child relationships are normally framed.

Traditionally, parents speak for and on behalf of their children and powerful professionals impose their realities on them (Chambers 1997). The decisions adults make, which they believe to be in the best interest of young people, are often protectionist in manner and based on their own realities. The decisions are made from

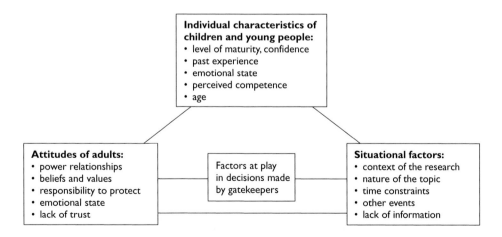

Figure 13.1 Factors affecting the attitudes of gatekeepers towards enabling young people to participate in research projects.

the viewpoint of the more powerful adult, power invested in them as part of society's hierarchical structure. The usual power relationship between adults and young people is captured well by Rowe (1991: 159) who defines power as 'the right to define how others should define'. This perceived power that adults hold over young people leads them to believe that they know more than children and that they understand the needs of children without having to ask them. In other words, adults know best. Thus, adults always know what is 'in the best interests of the child' and, therefore, it does not matter if the child's voice is not heard. Even if the child's voice is heard, it can safely be ignored because it can always be replaced by the more reliable adult source. Lee (2001) describes this as the 'silencing of children' and goes on to suggest that this view of children and childhood also gives adults reason to doubt whether children are even capable of speaking for themselves. Moving towards a more divested model of power, as described by Griffith (1996), requires adults to view young people as citizens and shift towards a more balanced power relationship. It requires adults to view young people not at the bottom of a hierarchy but as 'actors in a network of relationships' (Prout 2002: 74). Resistance to this shift exists though, especially among adults who fear giving any control or power to young people lest it lead to disharmony and as Alderson (2000: 110) describes 'fearful visions of powerless but responsible adults and powerful and irresponsible children'. Even when adults affirm children's rights to be heard and taken seriously, they inevitably raise questions about children's competence to participate (Lee 1999).

It is quite possible that some of the gatekeepers I approached took a traditional view of their relationship with young people and, thus, were resistant to giving consent for the study or even allowing children a say in the decision. Consenting to their child's participation might possibly threaten the status quo of their relationship. That is not to say that they necessarily acted to be 'obstructive' but that they believed (based on their own realities) they should act in the best interests of children, the ultimate goal being to protect children, particularly young children. Parents/carers may be cautious because of their own responsibility towards their children, or may feel their child is not fully competent enough to participate. Other reasons for 'obstructing' the recruitment process may be down to the potentially sensitive nature of a project (Cree et al. 2002), time constraints (particularly in relation to busy professionals and parents), lack of clarity about the project and thus a tendency to err on the side of caution. Parents of sick children, particularly those with chronic or life-threatening illnesses, may be too emotionally involved to take an interest in the study. Dealing with unknown researchers may result in a lack of trust and, therefore, a reluctance to participate.

Accessing young people for research projects must, therefore, be well planned for within a project schedule. Time must be taken to build trusting relationships with all gatekeepers and to justify the potential usefulness of the research. This time invested in meeting with gatekeepers is usually well rewarded. Information sheets need to be clear, detailed yet concise and appropriate for the different audiences – including the young people. Sending information and letters directly to the young people can increase the chances that they will be able to participate in deciding whether or not to take part.

Degrees of participation

Lansdown (1995: 17) defines participation as 'the process of sharing in decisions which affect one's life and the life of the community in which one lives'. Participation is about being counted as a member of a community, of being a citizen. The United Nations Convention on the Rights of the Child 1989 makes it clear in Article 12 that:

> States parties shall ensure to the child who is capable of forming his or her own views the right to express those views freely in all matters affecting the child, the views of the child being given due weight in accordance with the age and maturity of the child.

This international treaty gives young people a voice and, at the same time, presupposes a more socially active role for them. It recognizes the role of young people as social actors and, consequently, their role as fellow citizens.

Participation does not mean the token involvement of young people. It is about finding ways of incorporating their views into decision making processes within the context of what is possible both institutionally and culturally. Many instances of initiatives that attempt to make young people's voices heard can be found in the literature (Chawla and Kjorholt 1996; Edwards 1996; Silverman et al. 1995; Doorbar 1995; Lightfoot et al. 1998) but often participation is reduced to tokenism, or to decoration as described by Hart (1992). When done badly, it can act against the interests of the child and suggest a low value being placed on the child's views (Phillips 2000). Expectations can be raised and then dashed leading to disillusionment and further isolation (Johnson 1996). When young people feel 'ignored, bored, put on the spot or talked about as if they were not there' (DoH 2000), it is unlikely that any benefits will accrue. Several models exist that describe different levels at which participation can take place (Hart 1992; Abrioux 1998; Chawla 2001; Treseder 1997; Shier 2001), from situations where adults initiate consultation and listen to young people, through to projects directly initiated by young people themselves. Chawla (2001) asks us to acknowledge that the form of participation that is most appropriate varies with the circumstances, and that in seeking to facilitate young people's participation, it is important to understand at what level it already occurs and build on the experiences that young people already have. Participation by young people in research is a relatively new phenomenon. It is evidenced by a considerable shift in methodological approaches from those that see children as 'objects of concern' and passive recipients of adult socialization towards those that acknowledge children as social actors in their own right and engage them as active participants in the research process (Christensen and James 2000). Although there are many examples of research with young people as respondents, few actually engage with young people as co-researchers in a participatory approach.

Participatory research is a process of systematic reflective enquiry where researchers and participants actively engage in collaboration (Bernard 2000). Participatory research projects are about not only the research findings but also a broader engagement between those who have power and those who do not (West 1996). It requires that adults be prepared to relinquish certain elements of control and power, allowing young people to develop skills and capacities (Johnson 1996). Using participatory research with young people ensures them a direct voice in their representation, acknowledging them as social actors competent to commentate on their own lives and for what they are now, not what they will become. Implementing participatory research with young people is not without its difficulties. It takes time and requires that adults and young people collaborate in an 'open-minded process' in which no one knows the outcome (Chawla and Kjorholt 1996: 43). The role of the researcher is very different to that taken in traditional research where the researcher is 'outside' and takes an 'objective' stance. In participatory research, the outsiders (researchers) and the insiders (young people) are partners, sharing and learning together. Participatory research requires the researcher to be a 'committed participant and learner' having a 'committed involvement rather than detachment' (Martin 1994: 125). Though the ultimate aim is for young people to actively take part in all stages of the research process, it is not always appropriate or possible for this to happen. The degree to which young people can, or want to, participate in a research project can vary throughout its duration, thus impacting on the role the researcher takes.

Roles in participatory research: balancing control and decision making

During my own project, I fulfilled all the functional roles for participatory research as described by Stoeker (1998) but to varying degrees at different stages. I acted as an 'animator', helping the young people to develop a sense that their issues were important. I was a 'community organizer', helping them to plan, act and evaluate, stimulating their ideas rather than imposing my ideas on them. I was a 'popular educator', facilitating learning about research methods, allowing them to discover for themselves. Lastly I was a 'researcher', contributing my knowledge of research and my research skills. In general, the whole of the project was based on a collaborative partnership, with shared decision making and control. The balance of decision making, initiation and control, however, varied at different stages of the project and my role as a researcher changed in relation to this balance.

At times, during the project, the balance of decision making, control and initiation lay with me. This was particularly evident during the first phase of the project as I planned the methodology and carried out individual interviews with the nine young people initially recruited. In keeping with the participatory approach, however, even at this stage the young people were enabled to make some decisions with regard to the time and venue for the interview and the use of participatory techniques during the interview. Later in the project, involving the group in data analysis required me to take the lead as I decided which data analysis tool to use, namely framework analysis, and initially controlled its use. My role here was particularly geared towards that of 'popular educator' as I needed to help them understand how to use the tool and work through the analysis.

As the project moved into the participatory phase, the balance of decision making, control and initiation began to shift towards the young people and my role began to change. From being a traditional researcher, an 'outsider', I began to be a committed participant taking on other roles as described by Stoeker (1998). The young people began to work as a group, initiating ideas, controlling activities and making decisions with me acting as 'animator' and 'community organizer'. The shift was not without its dilemmas. One of the underlying principles of participatory research is that the participants must control the process of defining the research question(s). This was essential, as the purpose of the study was to enable young people to take some ownership of the work and to explore their own ideas and views about quality. When young people are given the opportunity to set research questions/topics for themselves, researchers may find that these do not fit with the requirements set by organizations or funding bodies. Researchers must avoid, at all costs, vetoing the decisions young people make as this will demotivate and disempower them. To avoid this conflict, it is vital that the context and the purpose of the study, and its limits, are set as soon as possible. In our project we agreed boundaries, discussed expectations, roles and the possible consequences of diverging too far from the original topic. At the same time, we discussed the time limits of the project and the extent to which the young people thought they could commit themselves. Over a period of a couple of weeks, the young people's discussions led to the formulation of a number of new research questions and methods for collecting data. They made decisions about who they wanted to collect data from and how they wanted to do it, but they made those decisions with my advice and support.

Involving participants in data analysis and dissemination is vital in participatory research and no less important when working with young people. It is essential that young people be enabled to make judgements about the data they collect and to interpret the findings according to their own realities. This not only serves to validate the findings and give added value to research but also gives young people a sense of ownership of the findings. As the group became involved in data analysis, they began to take more control. During the analysis sessions, the group tried hard to interpret carefully and fully, making decisions about how to chart the data. They made decisions about completing the analysis, clear in their belief that 'we should do it' even suggesting giving up time at the weekend to do so. At the beginning of the project, they were participating in 'my' research but it gradually became 'their' project in the sense that they felt they owned the findings. They formulated their own recommendations and determined to whom they wanted the findings sent. Though I drafted a final report and leaflet for them, they wanted the final veto and also to be acknowledged as the authors.

Though the balance of decision making, initiation and control lay with the young people, there were times when I had to make some decisions about how to proceed, albeit with the agreement of the young people. With the best will in the world, there are situations where young people acting as co-researchers will have neither the time nor the inclination to deal with complex and lengthy negotiations with gatekeepers or participate in data collection activities. Acting as 'researcher', I took on board the plans for accessing further samples of young people, collecting data from a group of Year 9 students and publishing a questionnaire in a national journal. At times, I felt that I was taking too much control but the young people did not perceive this to be the case. At the end of the project, I asked them where they thought most control had been at different stages of the project. Generally they thought that control had been shared evenly but that control was with them when deciding how to disseminate the findings.

Evaluating the participatory process

Reflecting on the degree of participation achieved in a research project can enable researchers and young people to learn from the strengths and weaknesses. It is also important, however, to evaluate the effectiveness of the participatory process as this can provide us with an insight into how adults and young people can work together in participatory research. One way to do this is to rate the process against the characteristics of effective participation as identified by Chawla (2001). According to Chawla (2001: 12), these characteristics are indicators of 'respect for young people's dignity as persons, mutual respect among group members, access, and support for growing levels of competence'. Table 13.1 shows how these characteristics were used to evaluate the participatory process of the project.

Generally, the project was characterized by effective and positive participation but areas of weakness were identified. Acknowledging where these weaknesses are can

Table 13.1 Evaluating the participatory process

Characteristic of effective participation	Project evaluation
Were participants fairly selected?	Not really – due to problems with recruitment
Did young people and their families give their consent?	Yes
Were the young people able to freely choose to participate or decline?	Yes – consent checked at every meeting or opportunity
Was the project accessible in scheduling and location?	Yes – local school: time chosen by group
Were young people respected as human beings?	Yes (their view)
Was there a mutual respect among participants?	Yes (their view)
Did the young people support and encourage each other?	Not always (their view)
Did the young people	
• have real influence and responsibility?	Yes (their view)
• have a part in defining the goals of the research?	Yes (their view)
• play a role in decision making and accomplishing goals?	Yes (their view)
• have the necessary information to make informed decisions?	Yes (their view)
Were the young people helped to express their own views?	Yes (their view)
Was there a fair sharing of opportunities to be heard and contribute?	Mostly (their view)
Were there occasions for the graduated development of competence?	Yes (my observations)
Were the young people helped to engage in the issues they initiated?	Yes (their view and my observations)
Did the project result in tangible outcomes?	Yes
Was there transparency at all stages of decision making?	Yes
Did the young people understand all the reasons for the outcomes?	Mostly (their view)
Were there opportunities for critical reflection?	Not enough (my reflections)
Were there opportunities for evaluation?	Yes but not enough (my reflections)
Did participants deliberately negotiate differences in power?	Not explicitly
Did the young people benefit from the experience?	Yes to different degrees (their evidence)

Source: adapted from Chawla 2001

enable the researcher to consider how they can be minimized in future projects. An important weakness of the project was that insufficient time was given for the young people to critically reflect on their own participation and hence the benefits they have accrued. This could be remedied by encouraging them to keep diaries of their experience, and making time for discussion, review and debriefing at key stages of the project. The group also felt that they did not always encourage each other enough and that sometimes the quieter members did not have the chance to be heard. This raises an important consideration – each young person may be able to participate at different levels and to varying degrees. So it is necessary for researchers to ascertain what support each young person needs to be able to participate to the best of their ability. This reflects the concept of the 'zone of proximal development' as described by Vygotsky (1978), where young people can be enabled to reach higher levels of competence under the guidance of more knowledgeable adults or collaboration with more competent peers.

Conclusion

The experiences of this project have served to show that involving young people in participatory research is a complex activity that requires adults to be flexible, ready to negotiate and willing to give up some of the power that they would otherwise hold. It is quite possible for the decision making to be shared but at times taken on board by either the adults or the young people without compromising the overall commitment to participation. At the same time, it is possible for young people to initiate and control activities yet not necessarily be the main decision makers. Involving young people in NHS participatory research is about opening up opportunities to them for meaningful participation based on their own realities and enabling them to have a real impact on the way their care is managed and delivered. It is about building mutual respect and dialogue rather than imposing fixed structures for participation. It is necessary, however, for researchers to acknowledge that participatory research is not an easy option. It requires time, resources, commitment and perseverance. At the same time, young people must be able to make the choice to participate or not. Participation is a dynamic process in which children and adults have to adapt and change. The way forward demands that we do not overlook or ignore the possible difficulties inherent in involving children and young people in research but that we work to overcome them to promote the right of children and young people to participate.

References

Abrioux, E. (1998) 'Degrees of participation: a spherical model – the possibilities for girls in Kabul, Afghanistan', in V. Johnson, E. Ivan Smith, G. Gordon, P. Pridmore and P. Scott (eds) *Stepping Forward: Children and Young People's Participation in the Development Process*, London: Intermediate Technology Publications.

Alderson, P. (2000) *Young Children's Rights: Exploring Beliefs, Principles and Practice*, London: Jessica Kingsley.

Bernard, W.T. (2000) 'Participatory research as emancipatory method: challenges and opportunities', in D. Burton (ed.) *Research Training for Social Scientists*, London: Sage

Chambers, R. (1997) *Whose Reality Counts? Putting the First Last*, London: ITDG (Intermediate Technology Development Group) Publishing.

Chawla, L. (2001) 'Evaluating children's participation: seeking areas of consensus', *PLA Notes*, 42: 9–13, London: IIED.

Chawla, L. and Kjorholt, A.T. (1996) 'Children as special citizens', *PLA Notes*, 25, London: IIED.

Children and Young People's Unit (CYPU) (2000) *Tomorrow's Future: Building a Strategy for Children and Young People*, London: HMSO (available http://www.cypu.gov.uk/) (accessed 15 October 2004).

Children and Young People's Unit (CYPU) (2001) *Learning to Listen: Core Principles for the Involvement of Children and Young People*, London: CYPU.

Christensen, P. and James, A. (2000) *Research with Children: Perspectives and Practices*, London: Falmer Press.

Cohen, J. and Emmanuel, J. (1998) *Positive Participation: Consulting and Involving Young People in Health-related Work – A Planning and Training Resource*, London: Health Education Authority.

Cree, V., Kay, H. and Tisdall, K. (2002) 'Research with children: sharing the dilemmas', *Child and Family Social Work*, 7: 47–56.

Department of Health (1994) *The Evolution of Clinical Audit*, London: DoH.

Department of Health (1997) *The New NHS: Modern and Dependable*, London: DoH.

Department of Health (2000) *Young People's Participation: Quality Protects Research Briefing no. 3*, London: DoH.

Department of Health (2001) *Children's Taskforce: An Introduction*, London: HMSO.

Doorbar, P. (1995) *Children's Views of Health Care in Portsmouth and South East Hampshire*, Portsmouth: P and SE Hampshire Commission and P Doorbar and Associates.

Edwards, M. 1996) 'Institutionalising children's participation in development', *PLA Notes*, 25, London: IIED.

Eiser, C. (1993) *Growing Up with a Chronic Disease: The Impact on Children and their Families*, London: Jessica Kingsley.

Griffith, R. (1996) 'New powers for old: transforming power relationships', in M. John (ed.) *Children in our Charge: The Child's Right to Resources*, London: Jessica Kingsley.

Hart, R.A. (1992) *Children's Participation: From Tokenism to Citizenship*, Innocenti Essays no. 4, Florence, Italy: UNICEF.

Hek, G., Judd, M. and Moule, P. (1996) *Making Sense of Research: An Introduction for Nurses*, London: Cassell.

Hennessy, E. (1999) 'Children as service evaluators', *Child Psychology and Psychiatry Review*, 4 (4): 153–9.

Information Commissioners Office (1998) The Data Protection Act 1998 (available http://www.hmso.gov.uk/acts/acts1998/80029--l.htm#sch1) (accessed 15 October 2004).

Johnson, V. (1996) 'Starting a dialogue on children's participation', *PLA Notes*, 25, London: IIED.

Kelson, M. (1995) *Consumer Involvement Initiatives in Clinical Audit and Outcomes*, London: College of Health.

Kelson, M. (1997) *User Involvement: A Guide to Developing Effective User Involvement Strategies in the NHS*, London: College of Health.

Kirby, P. (1999) *Involving Young Researchers: How to Enable Young People to Design and Conduct Research*, London: Joseph Rowntree Foundation.

Lansdown, G. (1995) *Taking Part: Children's Participation in Decision Making*, London: Institue for Public Policy Research.

Lee, N. (1999) 'The challenge of childhood: distributions of childhood's ambiguity in adult institutions', *Childhood*, 6 (4): 455–74.

Lee, N. (2001) *Childhood and Society: Growing Up in an Age of Uncertainty*, Buckingham: Open University Press.

Lightfoot, J. and Sloper, P. (2001) *Involving Children and Young People with a Chronic Illness or Physical Disability in Local Decisions about Health Services Development. Phase One: Report on National Survey of Health Authorities and NHS Trusts*, DH 1786 1.01 York: Social Policy Research Unit, University of York.

Lightfoot, J., Wright, S. and Sloper, P. (1998) 'Supporting pupils in mainstream school with an illness or disability: young people's views', *Child: Care, Health and Development*, 25 (4): 267–83.

Martin, M. (1994) 'Developing a feminist participatory framework: evaluating the process', in B. Humphries and C. Trumen (eds) *Re-thinking Social Research*, Aldershot: Avebury.

Morris, J. (1998) *Don't Leave Us Out: Involving Disabled Children and Young People with Communication Impairments*, York: Joseph Rowntree Foundation.

National Children's Bureau (NCB) (2002) *Involving Young People in the Recruitment of Staff, Volunteers and Mentors*, London: NCB.

National Early Years Network (NEYN) (1996) *Never Too Young: How Young Children can Take Responsibility and Make Decisions*, London: NEYN and Save the Children.

NHS Executive (1996) *Patient Partnership: Building a Collaborative Strategy*, London: DoH.

NHS Executive (1999) *The Protection and Use of Patient Information*, Leeds: NHS Executive (available http://www.doh.gov.uk/confiden/pguid2.htm) (accessed 10 November 2000)

Phillips, B. (2000) 'The end of paternalism? Child beneficiary participation and project effectiveness', unpublished master's dissertation, Institute of Social Studies, The Hague.

Prout, J. (2002) 'Researching children as social actors: an introduction to the children 5–16 programme', *Children and Society*, 16: 67–76.

Rowe, D. (1991) *Wanting Everything: The Art of Happiness*, London: HarperCollins.

Save the Children (2002) *Participation: Spice it Up! Practical Tools for Engaging Children and Young People in Planning and Consultations*, Cardiff: Save the Children.

Shier, H. (2001) 'Pathways to participation: openings, opportunities and obligations', *Children and Society*, 15: 107–17.

Silverman, W., La Greca, A. and Wasserstein, S. (1995) 'What do children worry about? Worries and their relation to anxiety', *Child Development*, 66: 671–86.

Stoeker, R. (1998) *Are Academics Irrelevant? Roles for Scholars in Participatory Research* (available http://uac.rdp.utoledo.edu/comm-org/papers98/pr.htm) (accessed 14 January 2000).

Strobl, J., Cave, E. and Walley, T. (2000) 'Data protection legislation: interpretation and barriers to research', *British Medical Journal*, 321 (7265): 890, (available http://www.bmj.com/cgi/content/full/321/7265/890) (accessed 10 November 2000).

Treseder, P. (1997) *Empowering Children and Young People: Promoting Involvement in Decision Making*, London: Children's Rights Office/Save the Children.

Vygotsky, L. (1978) *Mind in Society*, Cambridge, MA: Harvard University Press.

Warrell, S. (2000) *Young People as Researchers: A Learning Resource Pack*, London: Save the Children.

West, A. (1996) 'Young people, participatory research and experiences of leaving care', *PLA Notes* no. 25, London: IIED.

Chapter 14

From rhetoric to reality

The involvement of children and young people with mental ill health in research

Julia Waldman

Introduction

The principled and practical reality of implementing user involvement in research when working with children and young people with mental health needs raises a number of interesting questions, challenges and dilemmas. This chapter addresses issues that emerged from the evaluation of an innovative multi-agency, multidisciplinary service for children and young people experiencing severe mental health, emotional and/or behaviour difficulties called the Southampton Behaviour Resource Service. It introduces a framework for understanding types of service user involvement and explores a range of strategies that were used to help turn rhetoric into reality. These strategies are explored in relation to three stages of research project activity:

- design
- delivery
- dissemination.

In particular, the chapter will detail the dissemination phase as this proved to be the stage at which it was possible to be the most creative for involving users. Ways in which structural and situational factors acted as inhibitors to the fulfilment of some of the participative aspirations of researchers are explored. The chapter concludes with a summary of some lessons learned from the evaluation study about involving young people who experience mental ill health in research activities, with suggestions for further development of this form of participation.

Principles underpinning the evaluation study design

The Southampton Behaviour Resource Service (SBRS) presented as a complex social experiment (Seashore et al. 1983) in which its complexity could be expressed in a number of ways, not least in the different perceptions of success held by stakeholders from Education, Health and Social Services. Fujimura (1997: 99) acknowledges in this context that 'constructing *doable* problems, or successful research projects, is an uncertain process'. Using pluralistic evaluation seemed to be a way of managing and acknowledging different stakeholder interests and Smith and Cantley's (1985) perspective thus informed the design of the study.

Rather than treating such diversity as problematic, pluralistic evaluation acknowledges, even gives central place to, the varying perspectives proffered by different parties within a particular initiative.

(Smith and Cantley 1985, cited in Fuller and Petch 1995: 42)

Powell (1997) argues that part of recognizing complexity theory (Byrne 1999) and a plurality of views involves perceiving the research as a process in which researchers and research participants are actively engaged. The researcher threads the connections between the various narratives and perspectives to provide a detailed and independent account of the development and impact of a new service. This process can directly contribute to the further development of that service (Noponen 1997).

A linear approach to evaluative research would adopt a model of data collection – reporting – service considers findings and develops action plan. The role of the researcher in this model is one of independent 'expert' and involves non-deviation from the research route prescribed at the start of the study. In clinical research trials, the need to adhere to standardized routines is imperative to the validity and replicability of the research findings (Donenberg et al. 1999). End points assign the time at which the research may become useful, for example in relation to reviews of intervention models (Sinclair 2000).

A participatory action research approach uses a more diffuse and looped approach that creates different opportunities for the research to influence practice and visa versa. Humphreys and Metcalfe (2000) argue that this is the most graphic aspect of the action research process. So it seemed appropriate to try and build in a formative approach to the evaluation findings feeding into service development the SBRS. There were some key underpinning values within the proposals submitted for the commissioned study:

- commitment to participatory principles in the design and delivery of the evaluation
- a focus on both process and outcomes in service implementation
- use of an action research stance that allows for evaluative activities to inform the ongoing development of SBRS, with the evaluator taking a position alongside service providers
- design of outputs and dissemination activities that offer ways of making the public face and the voice of the evaluation study inclusive of participants, including young people as service users.

In the evaluation study of the SBRS, this had implications for the planning of outputs from the study, reflected in the conceptualization of a dissemination phase. Using only interim and final reports and papers for academic conferences would be insufficient and inappropriate to reach and represent the range of research collaborators' interests and abilities. The research needed to be the product of shared aspirations and ideas and its results should also be accessible to all those who collaborated in its production (Fuller and Petch 1995; Vander Stoep et al. 1999; Hall 1996). It is this set of value-based aspects of the study to which the themes of this chapter relate closely as they represent the sharp end of the interface between research and operational practice.

Service context

The service context is also important to highlight. The SBRS works with small numbers of children and young people facing many challenges in their lives as a result of which they will have been in contact with a wide range of mainstream and specialist agencies before being referred to the SBRS. In many cases, their lives are somewhat chaotic, lack stability and subject to crisis. Their experiences may have engendered a degree of cynicism with regard to professional intervention. Unfortunately, for some young people involved in risky and self-harming behaviours, their right to protection, assessed by others, may be at odds with their liberty rights. Applying the principles of involvement in decision making, even in these difficult but all too common scenarios, should still be a priority. Freeman (1992) argues that there is nothing intrinsically wrong with paternalistic restrictions that aim to protect. They must, however, be justifiable. Whatever their situation, it was vital that the young people using the service were not ascribed negative labels but respected as 'young people first' (Alston et al. 1992; Mental Health Foundation 2001) with the same rights and potential as any group in society. For the purposes of the study, parents and non-professional carers were also identified as users of the SBRS given the systemic model underpinning service interventions (see Henggeler 1999).

Frameworks for user involvement

Having identified the principles underpinning the research and service context, this next section presents in brief a framework for understanding the different levels of participation by service users in the evaluation of the SBRS. User involvement in service design and delivery has been promoted significantly in the United Kingdom since the mid-1990s through public policy and legislation and increasingly also in research (Department of Health et al. 2000; Lister et al. 2003; Faulkner and Morris 2004).

Wiffin (2004) identifies different models of user involvement as either being based on a hierarchy or a continuum. Four levels of involvement are identified: information, consultation, participation and control. Similarly, work on user participation carried out by the Community Care Support Force in the early 1990s defined five types. These are not mutually exclusive:

- veto
- consultation
- involvement
- control
- campaigning.

These are used to inform discussion about each of the three 'D' stages of the evaluation study as described earlier.

Design stage

The development of the SBRS went through a number of manifestations before the operational structure was agreed. This was due to changing information about levels of central government funding (Department of Health Child and Adolescent Mental Health Innovations Grant) and associated timescales. The evaluation was commissioned before the service was up and running and this was very helpful for the researchers in terms of being able to explore organizational issues at an early stage but impacted on the possibilities of involving users in the initial evaluation design because there were no users at this stage. A research group was established with representation from the three statutory agencies. Members had a range of views about what the evaluation should address and agreement was reached that a mixed-method approach would be acceptable focusing upon both outcomes (hard and soft) and process issues associated with the special inter-agency, multidisciplinary nature of the service, which also combined a community and residential provision.

To gain approval for the study from the local health ethics committee, the research plan had to present unambiguously how data would be gathered. A positive aspect of the approval process was the endorsement provided for the staged approach to the development of outcomes and research questions. This included a consultation phase to inform the development of the later stages of the study, a phase that included consultation with young people, their parents and carers. Their views assisted with decisions regarding which outcomes to track, what areas were important to service satisfaction and how views in the future should be obtained. Interestingly there was not a greater preference to face-to-face contact than postal questionnaires, which user research by SURE (2004) also found.

The views of those who were interviewed in this phase contributed directly to the decision to use both interview and postal feedback questionnaires in the main phase of the study to give users choice and to facilitate access to young people who might have been, for example, in penal or health related provision in another county when feedback was to be sought. Young people in the residential unit also contributed to the design of the child friendly format of the form, but again using a consultative rather than an involvement approach. The researchers did request representation by users on the research group but other members did not feel this appropriate due to the technical nature of the meetings and whether in principle this was a positive step. Also, the evaluation study found that while the service espoused partnership at commissioning level the approach to service development had actually been traditional in terms of the key partners involved. User organizations or groups were not involved in the planning or development as part of the management and steering groups (Waldman et al. 2002a). So the research could not draw upon these types of fora for consultation or participation.

At this design stage and in the delivery and dissemination phases the option of 'veto' was very important to facilitate. In essence, this means young people having the choice to say no to participation in the research. For young people who are in public care and who are in crisis, adults frequently *make important decisions about the teenager's life and living arrangements that the young person has little control over* (Browne 1998). Young people with complex needs may express their use of veto nonverbally, for example by the use of silence or behaviour that is an expression of resistance. If other systems and procedures are not in place, it may be difficult, particularly for young people in residential care, to exercise a right to veto (e.g. see Chakrabati and Hill 2000; Levy and Kahan 1991).

In terms of the evaluation, veto was represented by the choice given to children, young people and their carers to participate in the study or not. Codes of ethics in research demand that primary consideration is given to needs of service users (Butler 2000). In reality, this is a fine judgement call by the researcher, who is attempting to balance participatory principles, a rights perspective that includes open access to information, and due care for individuals who may be under significant stress and see limited personal benefit in being a research 'collaborator' as opposed to a research subject (Beresford 2000). This dilemma is particularly significant in the context of the SBRS, which is working with young people in crisis, experiencing mental ill health, and who may have developmental impairments. A vital aspect of informed choice is that young people should have access to appropriate information and that the presentation of choice should be offered in a manner appropriate to the young person's individual situation and level of understanding.

In the SBRS, evaluation consent for each child and young person was required to take part in the research. It was decided to use staff to facilitate consent at the point of entry to the service and special forms were designed and approved by the local ethics committee. In line with participatory principles, it was felt that if a young person was perceived by members of staff to be able to give their informed consent, then this should be actively sought rather than just asking a parent to do so. Staff explained to each young person what the implications were of giving consent, emphasizing that this consent may be withdrawn at any stage, and provided written information about the study. The latter was designed specifically for young people and amended with their input.

Using this approach, it was expected that not all young people would give their consent and, given the powerlessness many SBRS users may feel about decisions affecting their life, the ability to be able to say 'no' to a professional was viewed as something positive. This, of course, exemplifies a tension for the researchers, who were keen both to gain access to as many service users' case details and views as possible, and to promote choice. They had to respect the wishes of young people if they chose not to opt in and give consent, although few did not give consent during the study period.

It was felt that by asking staff to discuss consent with service users, this would increase chances of obtaining their agreement. For young people entering the residential unit, the discussion formed part of the induction. Some staff in the community team, however, did not universally share the rationale for the procedure, to apply participatory principles. Dalrymple (1997) argues that organizations operate a variety of overt and covert mechanisms to deny young people their rights. While some service users might exercise their right to decline to participate in the research, others may welcome the opportunity to express their views, whether that is to offer positive or negative criticisms of the service.

Delivery stage

Meaningful participation is reliant on children and young people feeling that they have some sense of control about what is happening to them, a particular challenge for those involved in work shaped by statutory obligations such as child protection or mental health. To take some control in their use of services, young people and their carers need workers to take account of a number of things including:

- demonstration of core professional values
- an enabling organizational context
- the negotiation of the complex interplay of needs, rights and resources
- the issues in managing the autonomy and protection needs of service users
- the centrality of power in partnership approaches
- relationships based on trust and mutual respect.

(based on Braye and Preston-Shoot 1995)

The question of giving control to young people was limited within the evaluative context, although it is important to note that the process allowed for some control over what young people chose to feedback about the service, and in what manner. Personal construct theory (Kelly 1995) asserts that 'Individuals bring their own meanings to any situation'. By obtaining the views of young people alongside those of professionals' regarding service effectiveness, it offers the possibility for different meanings of the service 'story' to be shaped more inclusively. Although in research, the application of consistency is important in accessing views, it was also recognized that the needs experienced by the range of young people using the SBRS impacted on meeting this principle. For example, those with developmental delays or impairments may be able to express views and give information on some matters but not all those being explored within the evaluation. If a young person wanted to end an interview quickly, then their wishes needed to be respected. Within limits of health and safety for both the researcher and young person, there was also choice about the venue for interviews. In the study, the youngest child to give feedback was 8 years of age.

An area of contention in research concerns the question of payment or reward to users. There were many discussions about this in relation to accessing the views of children and young people using the SBRS. Given the high level of professional interest that they are subject to simply by being referred to the SBRS, it seemed important to acknowledge the research participation as different from other forms of professional contact and to be honest that taking part was benefiting the researchers and the service, not the young person. It would have been false claim-making to ascribe gains to the young person. So a decision was reached to offer a token gesture of thanks (£5) to those who took time to be interviewed or completed a feedback form, which were additional activities specific to the research. Users who had consented to allow the researchers to read case notes but who did not give additional time were not given this form of thanks. Again, there was an acknowledged tension for the researchers between keeping this latter group of users informed but being aware that many were overwhelmed with forms and professional intervention. By choosing not to be involved in the feedback process, they had given a message about not wanting more contact with the research. Again, traditionally, questionnaires reminders may be sent once or twice but in the context of the SBRS the researchers were sensitive to this being inappropriate in many individual cases as it could have been perceived as an unwelcome pressure.

Another interesting aspect of service provision impacted on adopting a model of user group facilitation during the first two phases. The nature of SBRS interventions is individualized. The ethos of the residential unit positively discourages perceptions of residents as having any form of shared group identity, as this is felt to be inappropriate to a child centred approach. This makes it difficult to generate collective forms of involvement, although this was achieved successfully in the dissemination stage.

Dissemination

The researchers were aware that a participatory approach had been patchy in the first two phases of work, although points at which it was possible had been taken advantage of. However, at the dissemination phase, there was an opportunity to be more innovative, systematic and directive about contributions by users; young people, their carers and staff. It was possible to extend opportunities for participation because, in part, users would be actively opting in and staff could identify those who were in a good or reasonably good state of health.

A variety of activities and outputs were incorporated in to the research plans that were intended to meet the needs of the wide audience of potential collaborators and other interested parties. Many were intended to be accessible to and involve service users. In addition to formal papers and briefings, these included:

- website as an information resource about the study
- multi-authored book
- papers at conferences
- joint workshops run with researcher and members of the team
- national conference at the end of the initial three-year funding period.

Website

A section was created on the site called 'front-line views' and individuals were approached via staff with whom they had a working alliance for contributions. Pieces of work by young people, parents and staff were put up on to the website (http://www.sws.soton.ac.uk/brs).

Multi-authored book

A great deal of time was invested in working with staff and users to produce individual or group contributions on a whole range of service issues. This was challenging for the researchers but the end product made a wonderful complement to the formal research report. Users were encouraged to contribute and size or style was not an issue. The final publication contained contributions from nearly 40 people (SBRS staff, children, young people and parents) ranging from long chapters and articles to 'boxed' viewpoints, reaching over 200 pages in total (Waldman et al. 2002b). This represented powerfully another way for researchers to facilitate participation, empowerment and advocacy.

National conference 'Forging Links'

The publication was launched at a national conference run at the end of the study period. For six months before the conference, the principal evaluator worked in partnership with staff and a group of young people to enable them to deliver a presentation (young people) and workshop (parents) at the conference. The planning work, although challenging at times, provided a collective, team-working experience for the young people that many had not been able to experience in school or informal social settings. The final presentation included audio, video within a PowerPoint presentation and direct contributions by young people, as well as a 'comic' distributed to the whole audience on the day. Staff also made a display of art and comments by young people. The researchers also bought a number of throwaway cameras for use by young people in the months before the conference to develop a photo display on the day, although this was less successful – in part, because young people seemed to like to take pictures of people they knew and in some cases this compromised their protection and the privacy of their subjects. The parents planned and ran a role-play based workshop, which evoked very positive responses. The young people and parents were all given a payment for their time (given that the other keynote speakers were paid). They also had the additional bonus of meeting the first team of Southampton Football Club as the conference was held in its stadium, which made it a truly memorable occasion for some.

This set of activities represented a form of campaigning promoting the needs and interest of the young people using the service. Reports and conference presentations provided by the researchers (some with SBRS staff) were also important outlets for promoting positive messages about young people using the SBRS and making recommendations for policy and practice responses.

A collective experience

This set of activities represented a form of campaigning promoting the needs and interest of the young people using the service. The planning work, although challenging at times, provided a collective, teamworking experience for the young people that many had not been able to experience in school of informal social settings. Reports and conference presentations provided by the researchers (some with SBRS staff) were also important outlets for promoting positive messages about young people using the SBRS and making recommendations for policy and practice responses.

Conclusion and key messages

This chapter has explored issues related to user involvement in research in the context of the development of an innovative multi-agency child and adolescent mental health service. It has explored the possibilities and limitations for involving users within the evaluation study and identified that with flexibility, commitment and sensitivity, it is possible to involve users, although service structures and individual factors can impinge on the levels of involvement that may be possible at different stages of research. The issues explored also identify that there are possible issues of role conflict for researchers. There can be a need to acknowledge and balance the sometimes competing roles of consultant, facilitator and advocate with that of the objective researcher.

It was identified that in this study, the dissemination phase in particular provided creative and practical ways of involving users, but that the starting point in the research process of informed consent is crucial in this service context. The achievements of the young people presented a powerful affirmation of adopting a strengths-based approach and believing in the potential of even those whose life experiences have done them a great disservice. These activities also provided leverage to the SBRS to consider the involvement of service users at a more strategic level. So the final messages for involving young people experiencing poor mental health in research are:

- Believe it is achievable.
- Allow lots of time and resources in research plans to do it.
- If one area of work is not very successful look for others.
- Be flexible.
- Financial thanks may be acceptable.
- If the research is linked to a service work in close partnership with staff who have developed relationships with young people.
- Focus upon young people's strengths and potential.

Acknowledgements

Co-researchers who contributed indirectly to this chapter are Angele Storey and Jackie Powell.

References

Alston, P., Parker, S. and Seymour, J. (eds) (1992) *Children, Rights and the Law*, Oxford: Clarendon.

Beresford, P. (2000) *Service Users' Knowledge and Social Work Theory: Conflict or Collaboration?*, ESRC Seminar series, Theorising Social Work: 1–12 (available http://www.nisw.org.uk/tswr/bersefordedinburgh.html) (accessed 15 October 2004).

Braye, S. and Preston-Shoot, M. (1995) *Empowering Practice in Social Care*, Buckingham: Open University Press.

Brechin, A. (2000) 'Introducing critical practice', in A. Brechin, H. Brown and M.A. Eby (eds) *Critical Practice in Health and Social Care*, London: Sage.

Brown, D. (1998) 'The relationship between problem disclosure, coping strategies and placement outcome in foster adolescents', *Journal of Adolescence*, 21: 585–97.

Butler, I. (2000) *A Code of Ethics for Social Work and Social Care Research*, ESRC Seminar series, Theorising Social Work: 1–12 (available http://www.nisw.org.uk/tswr/ianbutler.html) (accessed 15 October 2004).

Byrne, D. (1999) 'Complexity theory and social research', *Social Research Update*, 18, 1–6, University of Surrey (available http:www.soc.surrey.ac.uk/sru/SRU18.html) (accessed 10 March 2002).

Chakrabarti, M. and Hill, M. (eds) (2000) *Residential Child Care*, London: Jessica Kingsley.

Dalrymple, J. (1997) 'Advocacy', in D. Garratt, J. Roche and S. Tucker (eds) *Changing Experiences of Youth*, London: Sage.

Department of Health/research in practice/Making Research Count (2000) *Quality Protects Research Briefings: Young People and Participation*, London: DoH.

Donenberg, G., Lyons, J. and Howard, K. (1999) 'Clinical trials versus mental health services research', *Journal of Clinical Psychology*, 55 (9): 1135–46.

Faulkner, A. and Morris, B. (2004) *Research Governance Framework . . . Review of Key Initiatives to Support User Involvement at Different . . . Initiatives in the Context of Forensic Mental Health Services . . . The Expert Paper on User Involvement: Implications for Ethics* (available http://www.dh.gov.uk/assetRoot/04/02/10/23/04021023.ppt) (accessed 10 June 2004).

Freeman, M.D.A. (1992) 'Taking children's rights more seriously', *International Journal of Law and the Family*, 6 (2): 52–71.

Fuller, R. and Petch, A. (1995) *Practitioner Research*, Buckingham: Open University Press.

Fujimura, J. (1997) 'The molecular bandwagon in cancer research: where social worlds meet', in A.L. Strauss and J. Corbin (eds) *Grounded Theory in Practice*, London: Sage.

Hall, S. (1996) 'Reflexivity in emancipatory action research: illustrating the researcher's constitutiveness', in O. Zuber-Skerritt (ed.) *New Directions in Action Research*, London: Falmer Press.

Henggeler, S.W. (1999) 'Multisystemic therapy: an overview of clinical procedures, outcomes and policy implications', *Child Psychology and Psychiatry Review*, 4 (1): 2–10.

Humphreys, C. and Metcalfe, F. (2000) *Research Approaches for Practitioners: The Role of Action Research*, ESRC Seminar series, Theorising Social Work: 1–7 (available http://www.nisw.org.uk/tswr/humphreysmetcalfe.html) (accessed 5 June 2002).

Kelly, G.A. (1955) *The Psychology of Personal Constructs*, 1, New York: Norton.

Levy, A. and Kahan, B. (1991) *The Pindown Experience and the Protection of Children: The Report of the Staffordshire Child Care Inquiry 1990*, Stafford: Staffordshire County Council.

Lister, S., Mitchell, W., Sloper, P. and Roberts, K. (2003) 'Participation and partnerships in research: listening to the idea and experiences of a parent-carer', *International Journal of Social Research Methodology*, 6 (2): 159–65.

Mental Health Foundation (MHF) (2001) *Turned Upside Down*, London: MHF.

Noponen, H. (1997) 'Participatory monitoring and evaluation – a prototype internal learning system for livelihood and micro-credit programs', *Community Development Journal*, 32 (1): 30–48.

Powell, J. (1997) 'Researching social work and social care practices', in G. McKenzie, J. Powell and R. Usher (eds) *Understanding Social Research: Perspectives on Methodology and Practice*, London: Falmer Press.

Seashore, S., Lawler, E.E., Mirvis, P.H. and Cammann, C. (eds) (1983) *Assessing Organisational Change*, Toronto: John Wiley and Sons.

Sinclair, I. (2000) *Methods and Measurement in Evaluative Social Work*, ESRC Seminar series, Theorising Social Work: 1–11 (available http://www.nisw.org.uk/tswr/humphreysmetcalfe.html) (accessed 5 June 2002).

Smith, G. and Cantley, C. (1985) *Assessing Health Care: A Study in Organisational Evaluation*, Milton Keynes: Open University Press.

SURE (2004) *We Did It Our Way! Summary Report of the SURE Team's User-Controlled Research Project – 24th October 2001 to 30th June 2003*, Chelmsford: MACA Partners in Mental Health (available http://www.maca.org.uk/temp/SUREspreportspsummarysp1.pdf) (accessed 29 June 2004).

Vander Stoep, A., Williams, M., Jones, R., Green, L. and Trupin, E. (1999) 'Families as full research partners: what's in it for us?', *Journal of Behavioural Health Services and Research*, 26: 329–44.

Waldman, J., Powell, J. and Storey A. (2002a) *Final Report: Evaluation of Southampton Behaviour Resource Service*, Southampton: Division of Social Work Studies, University of Southampton.

Waldman, J., Powell, J. and Storey A. (eds) (2002b) *Perspectives from Research and Practice of the Southampton Behaviour Resource Service*, Southampton: Division of Social Work Studies, University of Southampton.

Wiffin, J. (2004) *Beyond Listening: Involving Service Users*, PowerPoint presentation, Luton: Making Research Count (available http://www2.warwick.ac.uk/fac/soc/shss/mrc/userinvolvement/wiffin.ppt) (accessed 15 June 2004).

Chapter 15

Strategies for involving service users in outcomes focused research

Hannah Morgan and Jennifer Harris

Introduction

This chapter details the attempts of the authors to develop meaningful involvement with service users in a project that researched the development and utility of an outcome focus in assessment and review work with disabled adults of working age. The strategies employed are discussed within the context of wider debates about disability research, the influence of the funding agency and resource constraints.

The development of a social barriers/model understanding of disability, initially by disabled activists (Union of the Physically Impaired Against Segregation (UPIAS) 1976) and latterly by academics (Oliver 1983; Barnes 1991) has challenged the traditional notion that impairment – whether physical, sensory or cognitive – was the main factor in the disadvantages experienced by disabled people. Therefore, barriers rather than impairment are a more appropriate focus of disability research. Furthermore, research based on individual or medical understandings of disability was recognized as contributing to this process of disablement by perpetuating an understanding of disability as individual limitation causing disadvantage.

This has led to the charge that disability research is often a 'rip-off' (Oliver 1992), expecting the participation of disabled people as passive subjects without any real benefit for disabled people, either individually or collectively.

> Disabled people have come to see research as a violation of their experience, as irrelevant to their needs and as failing to improve their material circumstances and quality of life.
>
> (Oliver 1992: 105)

There has been considerable discussion within disability studies and more widely about the emancipatory potential of research to illuminate, challenge and remove disabling barriers including the development of an emancipatory research paradigm (Oliver 1992) and the articulation of its key principles (Stone and Priestley 1996; Barnes 2004). Simply put: 'Emancipatory research is about the systematic demystification of the structures and processes which create disability' (Barnes 1992: 122).

Emancipatory research is an epistemological approach to research rather than a methodology, and the principles that underlie it can be summarized as adherence to a social model perspective, accountability to disabled people and their organizations, and a commitment to producing research that is empowering both in its process and its outcomes (Barnes 2004). At the heart of emancipatory research is a rejection of the positioning of the researcher as an objective neutral participant in the research process. Instead, considerable attention is paid to the social relations of research production with the recognition that the emancipatory potential of research is determined by the extent to which disabled people (and other oppressed groups) are 'actively involved in determining the aims, methods and uses of research' (Zarb 1997: 52). It is vital that the social relations of research production are transparent and that it is clear where power resides and how it is being utilized.

The challenge for those of us undertaking disability research with a commitment to a social model of disability is how we seek to adhere to these principles within existing confines, not least the precarious nature of contract research careers and the dominance of funding institutions in the field. This chapter draws upon the experience of the authors undertaking a specified project, discussing the strategies for involving service users employed within a wider context of confines and limitations. Consideration is given to the effectiveness of these strategies and the relative impact of external factors.

The context of the project

The Outcomes for Disabled Service Users project, currently ongoing with a three-year lifespan, is an innovation to research the development of outcome focused assessment and review processes in services for disabled people of working age. The project forms the first attempt to introduce a focus upon the outcomes that disabled people wish to see from social services. It is fully compliant with the core principles of the social model of disability and, as such, makes an important contribution to debates concerning the best means of identifying and achieving the types of service that disabled people aspire to receive. It is core funded through a government grant programme and sited within a British university. The project works with one Social Services Department's disability service, which is responsible for all services provided to people with physical and sensory impairments aged 18–65 years.

The research team, being wholly committed to a social model of disability (Oliver 1983), have striven to incorporate key features of the original model and later developments into the project at every opportunity. These include awareness of, and willingness to, address environmental and attitudinal barriers to service provision and user led (not service led) provision of services to disabled people. The latter is considered extremely innovative within the context of social service provision in the United Kingdom. There is also wholehearted commitment to involving service users in the research about services in creative and meaningful ways.

Confines and limitations of the project

Undertaking research that forms part of a wider programme of work necessitates adherence to guidelines and codes of practice that are inherent to the programme, but which do not necessarily chime well with the ideals of researchers or practice within the field. Research conducted with disabled adults is often (as in our case) conducted within the wider remit of adult social care, in which the main focus is on the requirements of older people and, to a lesser extent, informal carers. These latter fields of practice, being less politicized in the United Kingdom than in other areas of the world (notably the United States), do not, as a rule, conform to the tenets of the social model of disability and are less likely to recognize its importance. It is frequently difficult to summon sufficient tact in rejecting the terminology and patronising practices that are widespread within the field of social care with older people. These tensions also exist in social care provision for younger disabled people, because most Social Services budgets are committed to older people's services and where practitioners still work 'across the age boundaries' (under and over age 65). Thus inappropriate practice is often transferred from one group of service users to the other, despite the relevance of a social model perspective in practice with older people.

There are also considerable constraints exercised through the medium of the funders of the research. While the Department of Health is committed to 'user involvement' in research funded through the programme, the extent of direction and commitment to it is not explicitly expressed. As with all other aspects of research, the extent of commitment is generally expressed in terms of the financial resources allocated, and these must be kept within modest boundaries. Furthermore, as part of a larger long-term research programme there is less room for manoeuvre in terms of involving users in shaping the main aims and objectives of the project, as the main research aims and question had been predetermined as an earlier part of the programme. This inflexibility inevitably conflicts with both the political and philosophical commitments of the authors and creates tensions that must be managed within the confines of commissioned government research agendas.

Strategies for involving service users

Notwithstanding the constraints discussed above, the research team and the wider unit in which it is situated have a long-standing commitment to meaningful service user involvement in research (Heaton 2002; Lightfoot and Sloper 2003). Therefore, the project was able to build upon extensive experience of working collaboratively with disabled people and service users, and draw on existing relationships with organizations of disabled people and a developing pool of knowledge about good practice.

Project advisory group

In common with the other projects that constitute the Outcomes Programme, a project advisory group was established and a range of 'experts' invited to join. This included the research manager from the Coalition of Disabled People based in the partner local authority. The involvement of a grassroots organization of disabled people from the research locale was felt to be significant for a number of reasons. First, and perhaps most importantly, because the inclusion acknowledges the user perspective as equal in value to those of other (more traditional)'experts' in the research field, such as academics, policy customers and the voluntary sector. Furthermore, it allowed a representative user voice to be heard much more centrally and at an earlier stage in the research process. An additional benefit was the ability of a local organization of disabled people to have both a local and national perspective on policy developments and the research project.

The input to the project advisory group provided by the user representative was invaluable both in terms of assisting the general progress of the project but more specifically in advising the research term about methods and strategies for increasing the level and quality of user involvement, for example through introductions to other groups. Indeed, the relationship developed to such an extent between the research team and the disability organization that a joint bid for research funding from the Social Care Institute for Excellence was submitted. While the bid was unsuccessful, its significance lay in the lead role taken by the Coalition and the potential for a reciprocal working relationship to be established.

However, tensions emerged due to the difficult relationship between the organization of disabled people and the local authority and ultimately the representative withdrew his membership of the project advisory group. It was made clear this withdrawal was not related to either the content of research project or the activities of the research team, but rather the organization of disabled people felt that their continued involvement with the project might be construed as support of the more general activities of the Social Services Department with which they were at odds.

This turn of events illustrates the difficulties posed for researchers when seeking to balance the involvement of a range of stakeholders, particularly those who feel their credibility may be compromised by shared membership of an advisory group. On one level, it was frustrating for involvement to break down due to external factors after considerable effort had gone into developing the relationship. However, on the other hand, it gave the research team considerable insight into local relations, and in some senses should be seen as part and parcel of the challenge of increasing the meaningful engagement of often conflicting or even contradictory perspectives and stakeholders.

Service user panel

The 'usual' means of involving service users in research of this kind is to form a service user panel that meets two or perhaps three times a year to discuss the progress of the research and to give a steer on important issues. At the outset of the project, the researchers discussed this form of involvement and found it lacking in some important respects. First, our commitment to real and meaningful involvement meant that the constraints of meeting with service users only six times in three years would limit the amount of influence they could realistically exert over the decision making process. Second, there were very real concerns about how representative any small group of service users could be due to the huge geographical area covered by the research. The site includes affluent rural areas and pockets of extreme deprivation. The issue of representativeness also applied to inclusion of different impairment groups and other types of identity such as ethnicity, gender and age. It would be impossible to include service users from all impairment and other groups and, inevitably, the selection process would exclude many. Third, the huge geographical area would have implications on the willingness and ability of individual service users to travel to meetings. Again, a few people who either happened to live in one area or had access to transportation could dictate membership and influence. Furthermore, as suggested earlier, involvement has to be resourced within the financial constraints of the project and there were concerns that large chunks of the 'involvement' budget might be eaten up by transport and other access costs, thereby limiting the number of participants.

Bearing all these in mind, our strategy developed along the lines of 'lateral thinking', particularly in terms of developing better ways of utilizing limited resources to maximize both the quantity and the quality of involvement.

The 'virtual panel'

The first decision taken was to disband the idea of using any static formalized regular meeting process. This overcame most of the issues highlighted above, including geographical and transportation problems. Once this decision had been made, the task became how to set up a 'virtual panel' with fluid but inclusive boundaries. Thus, service users and disabled people (as either individuals or as organizations) could join, participate and leave at any stage of the life of the project (a conscious decision was taken to include disabled people who both used and did not currently use services). This had obvious advantages for many service users as well as for the project, since some issues are more interesting to some individuals than others, but also life circumstances and impairment effects (Thomas 1999) may dictate the extent of available personal energy and thus commitment that can be given to the work. Similar issues apply to organizations of disabled people and services users who are characterized by precarious funding and are, by and large, staffed by volunteers (Morgan et al. 2001).

Under the 'traditional' service user involvement design, the research team are in the driving seat, with service users playing an advisory role. This generally extends to the formalized meeting structure with agendas set in advance, usually by the research team. However, a decision was made that where face-to-face consultation and advice giving was necessary, it would be far better to seek to join groups already in existence, where the membership were in control of the agenda and decision making processes, and could set the terms of their involvement. This proved to be an important strategy in terms of the exercise of users' 'voice' and recognition of control issues. This type of consultation can be challenging for researchers as striving for greater equality in relationships between researchers and service users inevitably involves shifting power and control from the hands of the research team to reflect a more equitable balance. It means that issues about the research are not necessarily at the top of a disability group's agenda and that the priority given to particular aspects of discussions are determined by the membership in attendance, rather than the researcher. This can lead to tensions for researchers who may be under pressure to undertake consultation on certain issues at specific stages of the project when this does not tally with the priorities of the partner organization.

Flexibility also extends to the media of participation. Once the traditional structure was disbanded, it became possible to envisage new forms of participation, such as email lists for consultation on document content and postal participation. In the event, neither of these strategies were taken up by service users to any great extent, for reasons that were unclear, but which may have been to do with access to computer equipment in the former. It was also apparent that many of the groups involved appreciated face-to-face contact as it made it easier for them to exercise control and choice over the way in which information was exchanged, e.g. it allowed questions to be asked of the research team and issues explored in 'real time' rather than the more extended toing and froing of email or postal conversations. Face-to-face meetings also allowed a greater element of reciprocity in the relationship. Groups could tap into the specialist knowledge of the research team and exploit in a small way the contacts and resources of a research institute, for example through sharing information about recent research and policy developments.

However, the inclusion of such strategies allows for a much wider range of consultation, both for targeted and routine purposes, and is ultimately far more inclusive than traditional groups.

Developing accessible consultation

To maximize levels of involvement, it was felt important to pay considerable attention to developing accessible methods of communication. As a matter of routine, all project documents were made available in large print, electronically, in Braille and on tape. Due to resource constraints, it was not possible to routinely produce documents in community languages, although a commitment was made to production should it be requested. This was felt to be a reasonable compromise because there were only occasional instances of service users in the research locations requesting their social services documents in community languages compared to levels of requests for large print and other alternative formats. It was made clear on any project document that all efforts would be made to produce alternative formats if they were requested.

Any attempt to increase the quantity and quality of involvement and participation requires particular attention to be paid to the process of ensuring informed consent from participants. The project developed work already undertaken by the research unit on the development of clear and concise documents to enable participants to make informed decisions about their involvement (Heaton 2002). Considerable attention was paid to ensuring leaflets were clear and concise with an emphasis on plain English and demystifying the research process. Furthermore, it was decided to produce video versions of the leaflets. Two versions were produced. The first, in plain English and aimed at people with learning difficulties or with acquired hearing loss, was recorded by an actor and subsequently subtitled. The second, aimed at British Sign Language (BSL) users, was developed in consultation with a BSL tutor/consultant. While the research team had the advantage of having a member with considerable expertise in D/deaf research as well as being a BSL user it remained a difficult process to translate abstract English concepts into BSL.

Wider consultation

It was felt important that the project involved disabled people and their organizations more generally and service users at a national level as well as within the local authority. Therefore, at an early stage in the project a seminar was jointly organized with Shaping Our Lives, the national user network, to bring together service users, practitioners and academics to discuss their different perspectives on the utility of an outcomes focus in social service provision. The seminar built on the existing relationship between the research unit and Shaping Our Lives, who were also conducting outcomes focused research (Shaping Our Lives 1998, 2002).

The day stimulated lively discussion (Morgan and Harris 2002) and while disagreement remained about the way in which agreed outcomes are produced, the seminar was characterized by a respect for differing perspectives and recognition of the validity of the contribution from each participant. This kind of coming together of different stakeholders in research helps to make dialogue an ongoing process rather than something that solely occurs at particular stages in the research process. Participants are able to shape each other's thinking and gain access to views, perspectives and knowledge that they may not come into routine contact with otherwise. Furthermore, the involvement of representatives from funding agencies and policy customers means users, practitioners and researchers can influence the embryonic stages of research agenda development.

Conclusion

User involvement and consultation, whether in service development, provision and evaluation, or in research about services, is 'no longer simply a good thing' (Beresford 1992). It is required by legislation and policy guidance and demanded by service users and their organizations. This is supported by the articulation of a social model of disability, the evolution of critical disability studies and the development of an emancipatory paradigm in disability research. Increasing levels of involvement in all stages of the research process have been broadly welcomed by researchers as contributing to the validity and quality of the research produced and as a positive influence on the process of research and its impact on all participants.

However, consensus about the best ways of involving users and the manner in which this participation should be resourced has not yet been achieved. This frequently leaves researchers with the challenge of aspiring to meaningful engagement within contexts that may not be fully supportive of, or may even be counter to, this involvement. The most obvious of which are the levels of resources the major funding agencies are prepared to commit to involvement in particular projects. While levels have certainly increased in recent years and funding agencies are increasingly receptive to more creative methods, funding for involving service users outside the confines of particular projects remains constrained. Most research units, whether within or without higher education institutions, rarely have sufficient funding to involve users routinely in the development of research bids. This is compounded by the relative absence of service user voices in the genesis of research agendas and programmes. Thus, considerable effort needs to be directed at engaging service user perspectives at the macro-level of research production.

However, as we have suggested, much is possible at the micro-level or coalface of research production. Expertise is growing around the most effective ways of involving users at all stages of research and this can be seen as a cumulative process whereby user perspectives are increasingly 'internalized' by researchers, informing their thinking and practice. It is clear that negotiating new relationships and new ways of 'doing user involvement' can be a steep learning curve for all concerned and so the emphasis needs to be on learning from this process rather than feeling under pressure to get it right straight away.

References

Barnes, C. (1991) *Disabled People in Britain and Discrimination*, London: Hurst in association with the British Council of Organisations of Disabled People.

Barnes, C. (1992) 'Qualitative research: valuable or irrelevant?', *Disability, Handicap and Society*, 7 (2): 115–24.

Barnes, C. (2004) 'Reflections on doing emancipatory disability research', in J. Swain, S. French, C. Barnes and C. Thomas (eds) *Disabling Barriers – Enabling Environments*, 2nd edn, London: Sage.

Beresford, P. (1992) 'No longer simply a good thing', *Community Care*, 26 March supplement, ii.

Heaton, J. (2002) 'Informed consent in the "Time for Families" project', presentation to the Health and Social Care Group, Social Policy Research Unit, York, 17 September 2002.

Lightfoot, J. and Sloper, P. (2003) 'Having a say in health: involving young people with a chronic illness of physical disability in local health service development', *Children and Society*, 17: 277–90.

Morgan, H. and Harris, J. (2002) *Outcomes for Disabled Service Users: Service User and Professional Perspectives*, York: Social Policy Research Unit, University of York.

Morgan, H., Barnes, C. and Mercer, G. (2001) *Creating Independent Futures: Stage Two Report*, Leeds: Disability Press.

Oliver, M. (1983) *Social Work with Disabled People*, London: Macmillan.

Oliver, M. (1992) 'Changing the social relations of research production?', *Disability, Handicap and Society*, 7 (2): 101–14.

Shaping Our Lives (1998) *Shaping Our Lives Project Report*, London: Shaping Our Lives.

Shaping Our Lives (2002) *From Outset to Outcome: Report of Four Development Projects on User Defined Outcomes*, London: National Institute for Social Work.

Stone, E. and Priestley, M. (1996) 'Parasites, pawns and partners: disability research and the role of the non-disabled researcher', *British Journal of Sociology*, 47 (4): 699–716.

Thomas, C. (1999) *Female Forms: Experiencing and Understanding Disability*, Buckingham: Open University Press.

Union of the Physically Impaired Against Segregation (UPIAS) (1976) *Fundamental Principles of Disability*, London: UPIAS.

Zarb, G. (1997) 'Researching disabling barriers', in C. Barnes and G. Mercer (eds) *Doing Disability Research*, Leeds: Disability Press.

Chapter 16

Working with older women in research

Benefits and challenges of involvement

Lorna Warren and Joanne Cook

Introduction

Despite the growing political and research interest in user involvement (Kemshall and Littlechild 2000), detailed and critical accounts of projects working with older people based on the direct experiences of people who took part are still relatively scarce (Warren and Maltby 2000). This chapter assesses the background to, and processes and outcomes of, involvement in research through the experiences of women aged 50+ from a range of communities who participated in the Sheffield-based Older Women's Lives and Voices: Participation and Policy in Sheffield (OWLV) project. The main focus is on a small group of volunteer researchers, recruited from the project participants, who worked with the academic researchers in carrying out one-to-one life story interviews with the remaining older women participants. The chapter considers aspects of training, interviewing, and dissemination activities, and their subsequent impact on the research design of the project as well as the entire project team. Highlighted are opportunities and limitations shaping involvement of this nature, and the contribution it can make to both the development of methods and the quality of findings is critically assessed.

It is important to note that, recognizing arguments about its neutrality and inclusivity (Thornton 2000), we favour the word 'involvement', especially when talking of our activities in working *with* older women in the research process. However, the OWLV project was set up to explore 'participation' within a broader theoretical and political framework, and we, therefore, also define and use this term (as outlined below). The older women in the project used the terms interchangeably, and quotes from them demonstrate the importance of context in debates about terminology.

Background

Developments in user involvement

A key aim of New Labour's modernization agenda is to tackle the limited extent of public involvement in local government and decision-making (Department of Health 1998; Cabinet Office 1999). Health and community care policies have been at the forefront in declaring empowerment *the* driving force within public services (Department of Health 1991). Increased participation and person-centred approaches (Nolan 2000) are intended to achieve more responsive and sensitive services and more legitimate and accountable public policies in light of demographic trends (Barnes 1997). Publications have aimed to change attitudes to, and practice in, the involvement of local people (NHS et al. 1998), with immediate implications for older people, who are the main users of those services.

Indeed, in 1998, the 'flagship' Better Government for Older People (BGOP) programme was launched with the goal of improving services for older people 'by better meeting their needs, listening to their views and encouraging and recognizing their contribution' (BGOP 1999). The associated 'learning network' (Department of Social Security 1998) has included an Older People's Reference Group to advise on the Department of Health's National Service Frameworks, and the joining up of lessons and recommendations for future action from the BGOP Older People's Advisory Group (BGOP 1999). The launch of Link-Age in August 2004 appears to be the latest phase in the aim to modernize and improve partnership working between services for older people.[1]

Alongside trends in the UK policy arena, the research arena has seen a growing interest in 'empowering strategies' within research (Bowes 1996). Critical perspectives from researchers, who are themselves disabled or users of services, and movements of disabled people and social care users, have highlighted the potentially disempowering nature of traditional academic research. Along with bodies such as the Centre for Social Action, they have developed alternative approaches to researching service users' lives and experiences (Beresford 1997; Centre for Social Action 1999). Increasingly, major funders of policy research, most notably, the Joseph Rowntree Foundation,[2] are promoting specific programmes of work with, as well as about, older people (Carter and Beresford 2000; Older People's Steering Group 2004).

Limitations to developments

Reports from the BGOP programme provide some evidence that engaging with older people will lead to services that are better tailored to meet their needs (BGOP 2000b; Hayden and Boaz 2000). However, the two-year lifetime of the BGOP pilots is an inadequate amount of time to systematically explore and evaluate user involvement, and details of older people's participation remain vague and questionable (Williams 2004). Despite some innovatory approaches, such as visioning techniques, older people's views seem to have been gathered most commonly in 'consultation' exercises (Boaz and Hayden 2000). Participatory initiatives tend to have a precarious existence and there is a 'glass ceiling' on subsequent involvement in developing a joined-up strategy (Older People's Steering Group 2004). The comments of the BGOP (2000a) Advisory Group raise additional questions about the effectiveness of consultation in involving older people who live in deprived communities, who have mental health problems or who are from black and other minority ethnic groups. It is still too early to judge whether this issue may be addressed within Link-Age by the remit of the Social Exclusion Unit (SEU) to improve of quality of life and inclusion of excluded older people in user-driven services.

It may well be that wider trends encouraging the involvement of users will ultimately have a more direct impact on the participation of older people in research and policy making. The call for 'evidence-based practice' in health care services

(Department of Health 1997, 1998, 1999, 2000), for example, resulted in the setting up of a Support Unit Consumers in NHS Research. Now renamed INVOLVE,[3] the unit has published guidelines for researchers and 'consumers' (*sic*) on involvement in research and development in the National Health Service (Hanley et al. 2003; Royle et al. 2001). Yet, evidence suggests that training for service users interested in being involved is still not readily available (Lockey et al. 2004). Much of the existing government department-funded research involving older people arguably remains driven by concern for 'best value' as much as quality of life and local democracy (Rappert 1997).

More independent and creative participatory initiatives are typically small-scale and supported by limited funding (Warren and Maltby 2000) or do not prioritize age as a primary focus (cf. The Toronto Group).[4] While older people have participated in research process in various roles (see Barnes 1999; Fisk 1997; Peace 1999; Thornton and Tozer 1994, 1995; Tozer and Thornton 1995), detailed and reflective accounts of their involvement are still scarce.

The Older Women's Lives and Voices project

Project background and aims

The OWLV project was shaped by ongoing debates and developments in user involvement. Our goal was to increase knowledge and awareness of factors shaping the quality of life of older women across different ethnic groups and their desire and ability to have a say in the services which are available to them (Cook et al. 2004). The relatively few qualitative UK research studies that have focused on the lives of older women have commonly marginalized the issue of ethnicity (cf. Bernard et al. 2000) and remained focused on the problems of later life (Wray 2003). We wanted to explore the impact on older women's lives of the intersection of ageism, sexism and racism but we wanted to do this without treating older women as passive victims or, in terms of research and policy making processes, 'quiet voices' (Barnes and Bennett 1998).

As social gerontologists, we were supportive of the theoretical shift in emphasis on dependence and senescence to one on 'participatory', 'active' or 'productive ageing' (Walker and Maltby 1997). However, we were aware of the elusive and contested nature of notions of participation and empowerment within a welfare context (Counsel and Care 1994). Welfare provision tends to draw from consumer models of involvement rather than user empowerment models based on clearly defined rights (Barnes and Walker 1996). An 'evolving process' (Stevenson and Parsloe 1993), involvement may be characterized by a number of obstacles for older women (Hobman 1994; Walker 1998; Warren 1999). Summarized here, they include:

- the pervasiveness of stereotypes applied to older women
- their lack of effective sanctions
- their political passivity due to culturally designated informal caring roles
- their absence from formal economic structures and institutions: key sources of political consciousness and channels of representation.

Where women have been involved in organizations, their demands and issues (particularly relating to health and welfare) have typically

- taken second place to those of male pensioners or of younger women (Curtis 1995; Sharpe 1995)
- omitted the experiences of black and minority ethnic women (Hooks 1986; Butt and Mirza 1996; Patel 1993).

In relation to local governance, then, older women display low levels of 'politeracy' and 'moralicity', and their position at the margins of political activity is especially characteristic of black and minority ethnic women (Curtis 1993; Simney 1998; Newman 2001). Given this picture, as feminist researchers committed to social equality, we wished to take a partnership approach to the project, involving older women as citizens and potential service users, not just as service users (Thornton 2000). This meant finding ways for older women to be involved in designing, carrying out and promoting the research, in the process 'demystifying' their lives as a basis for change (Reinharz 1992).

Project methods

We decided upon a mix of methods: discussion groups, life story interviews and a video. Elements of these methods have already been discussed in previous publications (Cook et al. 2004; Warren et al. 2003). Here, we concentrate on a small group of older women researchers who worked with us in carrying out one-to-one life story interviews with the other older women participants in the project, considering aspects of training, interviewing, and dissemination activities.

The older women researchers were recruited from the discussion groups that we ran at the first stage of the project with 100 older women, aged 50–94 years. Participants were from White British, Black Caribbean, Chinese, Irish and Somali communities, approached through existing social groups and political forums in Sheffield. We explained to the women in the groups that we had two goals for the second stage of the project:

- to find out in more detail through individual life story interviews about the issues they had identified as being of importance to their quality of life, including their desire and ability to have a say about these issues
- to work with a small number of older women themselves in carrying out these interviews.

Of influence on the design of the second stage, especially, was Barnes' (2002) observations on the limitations of 'mainstream' theory and practice (her own included) in user participation in their failure to accommodate emotional experience, story-telling and diverse debates, as well as to develop more creative ways of working. We chose a life story approach because of its potential to illuminate the 'inner' side of ageing at the same time as giving people agency in defining their own needs (Plummer 1990; Ruth and Kenyon 1996; Hazan 1994). We wanted to recruit older women to interview other older women because we could find no examples of where it had been done before using a relatively unstructured format. It also gave us the chance to explore whether a greater parity of age and, where possible, ethnic background between interviewer and interviewee had an impact on the telling of individual stories. By featuring older women centrally in both process and end result, the making of the project video represented further efforts to share 'responsibility' and control (Bowes 1996; Barnes 1999).

Ten older women from the discussion groups expressed interest in working with us as researchers though, over time, the group was reduced in number to eight due to health reasons and the sad and unexpected death of one member, Ying Wah Cheng. The remaining members, who stayed with the project until its completion, comprised Norma Clarke, Pat Hadfield, Pam Haywood-Reed, Lilleth Millen, Movania Parkinson, Judy Robinson, Jean Wilkinson and Winnie Winfield. They became known collectively as the volunteer (as opposed to academic) researchers or 'the volunteers', for short. Their ages ranged from 50 to 86 years, slightly more coming from working class compared with middle class households. Notably, there was no volunteer from the Somali groups, whose members uniformly were non-English speaking.

Working with the volunteers

Training

Aspects identified as crucial to older people's successful involvement in research include developing confidence to learn new skills, adequate training, and attending to practical arrangements (Barnes and Bennett-Emslie 1997; Cormie and Warren 2001; Older People's Steering Group 2004). To prepare for joint working, the volunteers took part in a series of workshops. These were typically half-day events, incorporating transport, refreshments and lunch, and university-based though, on a couple of occasions, we used a comfortable and accessible community centre, central to the city, as the venue.

We were aware of debates concerning payment for individuals actively contributing to problem solving. However, our study was an independent exploration rather than a directly consultative or co-productive exercise between older women and service purchasers and providers. Our compromise was to recognize the contribution of the older volunteer researchers by offering them an honorarium payment for their involvement.

The training covered research design, interviewing, basic analysis, and presentation and dissemination activities. Five workshops were run as planned. The first provided the volunteers with the opportunity to get to know each other and the academic researchers better, to share the reasons why they volunteered, what they hoped to get out of taking part, any concerns they had – especially ethical – about interviewing, and what skills they might bring to the interview process. The session helped to build confidence as well as to identify the main issues in supporting the volunteers.

In the second workshop, a summary of findings from the discussion groups was taken, alongside the volunteers' own experiences, as the basis for the research team as a whole to identify key themes underpinning older women's quality of life and expectations and experiences of having a say. These themes were then used to develop a checklist of questions or aide-memoire (Booth and Booth 1998), to guide the life story interviews, which were designed chiefly as 'conversation with a purpose' (Burgess 1984). The volunteers were also introduced to the film crew, opening discussions on how to proceed with the making of the project video.

In the third workshop, the volunteers were acquainted with practicalities and experiences of carrying out interviews. In the first part of the session, the academic researchers demonstrated interview techniques, inviting the volunteers to identify examples of good and bad practice. The volunteers then practised interviewing in groups, taking it in turns to play the respective roles of interviewer, interviewee and observer/commentator. As part of the exercise, they tested the workability of the aide-memoire, fine tuning wording, questions and prompts as they went along. They also familiarized themselves with the processes of setting up interviews, using tape recorders, attending to ethical issues, including obtaining interviewee consent for taking part in the project, ending interviews and submitting interview tapes. A raft of associated guideline documents subsequently accompanied this session, forming a 'interview pack'.

The fourth workshop constituted a feedback session. Approximately half-way into the life story period, volunteers were invited to give their perspectives on the effectiveness of the aide-memoire and of life story interviews, the content of interviews, and practical and personal experiences of interviewing.

We had originally envisaged devoting the fifth and last of the timetabled workshops to activities leading to dissemination of the project findings. The main intention was to invite comments and feedback on the codings we had used for the interview data and the key themes subsequently identified. However, it was at this point that we were forced to recognize two issues:

- the volunteers' desire to be more fully involved in preparing for and presenting the findings from the study, especially at the planned seminar for a local audience of older people, policy makers, service providers, professionals and academics
- the subsequent insufficiency of the agenda to meet the training needs of the volunteers.

As a result, the fifth workshop developed a new agenda of activities that included:

- group discussion on the wider experience of working as volunteer researchers
- arranging interviews with the academic researchers team on their motivations for and experiences of joint working with older women
- planning for a jointly written edition of the project newsletter
- discussion with the head of filming on the editing of the OWLV video.

In addition, four extra workshops were run to develop skills in basic analysis and joint writing, as well as to prepare for the seminar, bringing the final total to nine training sessions. These proved to be particularly intensive sessions in which, among other things, the volunteers:

- were introduced to the basic principles of qualitative data analysis using computer software (in this case, QSR NUD*IST 4)

- discussed and debated codings of the interview transcripts and emergent themes
- produced poems and short written reflections on their experiences (cf. Warren et al. 2003)
- team-edited presentation scripts
- helped to decide on the venue, agenda, format and practical arrangements for the seminar
- rehearsed for the seminar presentation.

Interviewing

Issues of confidentiality were a dominant aspect of training for the volunteers. Respect for confidentiality constituted a primary ground rule for the life story interviews, which is why we gave all older women willing to be interviewed the chance to select their interviewer in person. The uniform preference for the Somali older women was to be interviewed by one of the researchers working with an 'outside' interpreter. This was a reflection of cultural norms of privacy and the women's desire to keep issues in their lives hidden from members of the local community. As a result, the absence of a Somali volunteer did not directly disadvantage older women in the Somali groups.

A translator working with one of the academic researchers was also arranged for half of the life story interviews with members of the Chinese discussion groups. However, in this case, where women were participants were geographically dispersed throughout the city, privacy was not an issue. A translator was needed primarily because Ying Wah Cheng was the sole Chinese volunteer (see Warren et al. 2003 for a brief discussion of issues involved in using translators in research). Issues of privacy raised by a small number of the White British groups were also respected, though other women preferred the idea of talking to someone they knew rather than to a stranger.

Ensuring that 'acceptable researcher/subject relationships' (Dingwall 1980: 876) were achieved within the life story interviews was also a priority. Commentators have debated the importance of dynamics of control (Cornwell 1984), communications skills (Richards 1994) and sympathetic treatment over parity of age (Barnes 1999). Concerns shared by all in the OWLV project related to the volunteers' credibility as witnesses and their reactions to respondents (Gearing and Dant 1990). Bearing in mind that one-off interviews or meetings are likely to place some limitations on participants 'telling all' (Bornat 1993: 41), the most obvious and least intrusive way to monitor encounters was, again, through thorough inspection of the interview transcripts. They showed variation across volunteers, chiefly in terms of interview length and confidence in prompting responses, but 'fruitful interviews' nevertheless, the importance lying in the attempt to reduce inequalities (Fisk 1997: 58).

Dissemination

It was uniformly recognized by the volunteers, especially having been shown what was involved in the coding of just two anonymized interview transcripts, that the detailed and intensive analysis of the OWLV data required a level of expert skills and experience that was unquestionably beyond the remit and resources of the project.

However, by working together to agree key themes, compose the presentation and identify workshop groups, the OWLV project seminar – held, not without some irony, at Sheffield United football ground in April 2002 – was developed in a way that captured the lives and priorities of the volunteers and the women they interviewed. The presentation was written in the women's own words and included their individual reflections on the experiences of being involved in research. Furthermore, the workshop groups were focused upon making progress with service providers and other researchers to try to develop ways of working together in the future and of extending the involvement of older women in service decision making. As a result, we were successful in getting local service providers to attend the seminar and at least listen to the voices of older women.

The role of the volunteers in dissemination did not stop there, however. They contributed to the project newsletters and other publications (Warren et al. 2003). We made joint presentations at an ESRC Growing Older programme meeting, local and national seminars including the Toronto Group Research and Empowerment seminar series, and national conferences, including the 2002 annual conferences held by the British Society for Gerontology and INVOLVE respectively. We also ran specialist local seminars on involving older women in research in Birmingham, Liverpool and Sheffield as well as involving the volunteers in research-led teaching at Sheffield University.

All aspects of the volunteers' involvement – including their involvement in wider community activities – were filmed for a video of the project.[5] The making of the video required the drawing up of consent forms and ground rules on filming etiquette before the volunteers could engage in discussion about the topics they wished to cover on film and material to be edited and cut. In the absence of a Somali researcher, two nominated spokeswomen were filmed as representatives of the views of the group members while the translators chosen to compile the Somali and Chinese versions of the videos had worked closely in development activities with the respective groups.

Outcomes of involvement

In these remaining sections, we explore the benefits and limitations of involving users in this study. In doing so, we draw upon analysis of the video tapes from two of the training sessions with the volunteers and feedback notes from the other training sessions, a discussion group with volunteers on their experience of involvement, and the presentation on involving older women in research written jointly by the research team and the volunteers.

Outcomes of involvement for users and potential users of services need to be assessed, among other things, in relation to reasons for becoming involved. Research, based on a sample of younger (34–44 years) White British women has shown that seeing yourself as 'someone who gets involved' is by far the most positive predictor of participation of any kind of collective action by women. However, identifying with other women, a sense of getting a bad deal in society compared to men, and the belief that individuals can have an impact on change also matter (Kelly and Breinlinger 1995).

The volunteers did, indeed, typically come from a limited number of the more politicized groups and were among the younger and most vocal respondents in these groups and/or already active in public or voluntary roles. It was notable, if not surprising, that participants in the discussion group who did not want or feel able to be involved in the research as volunteer interviewers voiced reasons that included confidence, language, literacy, health, energy, as well as alternative interests and commitments. The failure to recruit a volunteer from the Somali groups was primarily due to language barriers but may also have indicated other perceived barriers preventing Somali women from identifying with the volunteer group.

Indeed, there were differences among the volunteers in experiences relating to education, employment and migration, as well as in terms of cultural backgrounds. One volunteer had worked as a lecturer, for example, while another had spent much of her life at home, caring for her disabled son. The reasons for becoming involved in the project were various and included building confidence, gaining a voice, working with others to achieve shared aims, learning from others, and generating a better understanding of older women's lives and of the raw deal they face despite a lifetime of experience. The outcomes of their involvement were not always quantifiable or easy to measure or anticipate during the early design of the research. Here we offer examples at three levels: the individual, the collective and the research level.

Intrinsic and personal gains

One of the key benefits of involvement emphasized by the volunteers was that of breaking down isolation: understanding that they were not alone and that others were going through the same experiences of growing older. Providing the space for sharing experiences was a founding principle of the project, and the early days of the training sessions were no exception. The first stages of training sessions created the opportunity for women to listen to each other's life stories and develop connections and bonds. This process was essential to successfully building bridges and identifying the common ground between the different volunteers and the research team. The early training sessions developed research skills through encouraging the volunteers to draw upon their own experiences to develop specific and common issues that would be of concern to the women they were to interview. This was particularly well received. For example, the women talked of 'the sharing and the coming together', of 'feeling safe to talk, to open up and to share'.

Volunteers frequently spoke of how they 'valued the opportunity to hear the experiences of older women from different ethnic groups'. One volunteer expressed how:

> Regardless of differences, we are all women. Interviews with women from different ethnic groups isn't always different, there will be similar experiences common to being an older women.
>
> (Black Caribbean volunteer)

This process of shared learning was of benefit not only to the volunteers but also to the researchers: we were privileged to be part of it and to gain greater insight into the experiences of older women from working so closely with the volunteers.

Collective outcomes – voice and agency

While personal pleasure from being involved was a key motivation, equally as important was that the outcomes of their involvement reached beyond the value the volunteers gained for themselves. For all of the women, the process of getting the voices of older women reflected in the research and in local service provision was essential. The volunteers had not been involved in research before, they had little or no experience of researchers or service providers asking their views and had certainly never been involved in the development and application of a research project. Many of them spoke of:

> The importance of older women believing that they still have the ability to change their lives – to bring about changes.
>
> (Irish volunteer)

The difficulties were that past experiences could shape this belief:

> The women are talking about past experiences and still nothing has changed. Positive experiences and outcomes can shape this belief.
>
> (Irish volunteer)

This reflected views expressed in discussion groups with Somali older women who wanted reassurances that service providers would listen to them and that something would be done. They had been giving their views repeatedly for some time with no change or response from service providers.

One volunteer stressed the value she had derived from her involvement in the project:

> We can talk negative experiences but we need to turn these experiences into positive things . . . Sometimes we talk too much about the negative. If we remain isolated at home, we can lose sight of the positives. Bringing women together can create opportunities for sharing and working together for change.
>
> (Black Caribbean volunteer)

Another volunteer spoke of how:

> the people I interviewed felt that women of 50+ were not listened to at all, that this project was going to give them a voice and that changes might result – they found this wonderful.
>
> (Irish volunteer)

One notable outcome is that the women involved (both the volunteers and the members of the discussion groups) felt that they wanted to tell their life stories because it might be able to benefit others. In many cases, these others were the next generation of older women but emphasis was also upon getting service providers to listen. One volunteer aptly summed up key lessons that can be derived from these experiences:

[Through] older women coming together we can built our motivation, have a voice, feel valued, feel that we are important. We can also support each other at times of difficulty.

(Volunteer, discussion group transcript)

For some, working with other older women provided a source of positive role models and an increased belief in individual agency:

When I joined your project . . . I met different kinds of older women than myself: those who had a motivation and purpose that I did not have, an independence and self-worth which is not dependent on their serving their children or grandchildren. More than this, they became through their way of life a true inspiration to me. Participation has encouraged me to believe I can make a difference . . . Life is not over because my children are grownup: I can build a new life now and do new things.

(Irish volunteer)

These motivations for involvement illuminate some crucial lessons for researchers and policy makers alike: successful user involvement must provide the space for individual development, for shared learning and for building common ground. Equally, though, it has to provide research outcomes that reflect the experiences of the research participants and seek, to whatever degree possible, to carry these lessons into policy and practice.

Research benefits

The value of involving the older women volunteers can also be explored from the perspective of the research data and the contribution to the research process. One particular area where personal and research benefits overlapped was in training the volunteers to carry out the one-to-one life story interviews with members of the discussion groups.

The first set of training sessions, designed to develop research skills and to jointly write the aide-memoire, took a great degree of shared learning, negotiation and collaboration. The result was a more inclusive product than the research team could have achieved alone. The extensive discussions gave us the opportunity to debate with each other to ensure that the questions were not leading and to avoid assumptions about older women's lives. Many of the volunteers illustrated the gains they felt this approach had brought. One specific advantage related to being interviewed by another woman, and in particular another older woman:

When women get together, they often feel at ease. You can start with a question and its surprising how much you can cover if you feel at ease with one another. Being interviewed by another older women can be beneficial because we may have similar experiences and be sensitive around the issues raised.

(White British born volunteer)

Another volunteer commented:

> The answers I got back are those that, I feel as an older women, I could identify with their experiences.
>
> (White British born volunteer)

This sense of common ground and empathy did not, however, wipe away the nerves and make interviewing a simple process, as two other volunteers demonstrated:

> The day before I was nervous, thinking, why have I agreed to do this? The beginning was difficult because I was nervous. But, I enjoyed it and it went well. Obviously, how the interview goes depends upon how receptive the interviewee is and the dynamic between the two people.
>
> (Volunteer, discussion group transcript)

> I was nervous and a bit unsettled when interviewing. I was worried whether the information was what was needed.
>
> (White British born volunteer)

All of the volunteers were interviewed as part of the research and their reflections of this process revealed some benefits that, as researchers, we are not always aware of:

> For my own interview, I was sceptical of whether I had much of a life history to tell. I learnt a lot from being interviewed about myself.
>
> (Volunteer, discussion group transcript)

The interviewers felt they gained a great deal of insight from listening to their interviewees' life stories and they worked hard in the dissemination phases to highlight what they had learnt. Many of the women they interviewed had very different experiences to themselves. One volunteer expressed how:

> The interviews gave me the opportunity to learn and see the other side of things. I was surprised by some of the things that people did tell me. I felt privileged that someone I had just met told me this and trusted me enough to share their life stories. Often we carried on chatting after the interview had finished.
>
> (White British born volunteer)

Others also expressed how:

> It was reassuring to hear other women's experiences and to be able to say – well, that's how I feel.
>
> (Volunteer, discussion group transcript)

The project gained substantially from working in this in-depth way with the nine older women volunteers, and much of this was reflected in the rich quality of the data. For both the researchers and the volunteers, listening to older women's life stories broke down generalisation about what older women do, how they feel and what they want and desire. By implication, they also effectively challenged assumptions that may be made about the ability of older women, often classed with others as 'inarticulate subjects' to effectively engage in processes of research or policy making with lessons for researchers, policy makers and service providers alike (Booth and Booth 1996; Older People's Steering Group 2004).

Challenges to involvement

The OWLV project demonstrated the clear ability of older women to work together, pooling their experiences to develop a complex research agenda and inclusive research approaches. Researchers, policy makers and service providers alike could learn from these experiences and use similar methods to develop user involvement. The requirement to work in different ways, and with limited resources, is the real barrier to effective user involvement. Importantly, developing a participatory strategy requires time, money, commitment, flexibility, and the building of confidence and trust.

One of the fundamental constraints upon involvement is the duration and resources needed to involve older women in research in a meaningful and substantive way. This can sometimes double the costs of a research project, and so much time can be involved in recruitment and training that even when budgets have tried to take account of this they result in overrunning. Our need to provide extra workshops for the volunteers is an example of this. While the benefits of extending the volunteers' involvement were great, this meant continuing to run meetings and work together after the funds for the project had ended.

This led onto another major difficulty of partnership approaches to research: the issue of when and how to withdraw from involvement. Working in this partnership way raised expectations among the core group of volunteers. Since we have been unable to apply for funding to extend the project, many of the skills and bonds built up have been lost and the potential they offer underutilized. Consequently, it is fundamental to have a contingency plan so that groups who develop participatory research skills can continue to work together and also to take on a bigger role in the analysis and dissemination of findings. For example, the volunteers wanted to be involved in the analysis of the life story interviews and in other stages of interviewing, such service provider interviews. The funds for this were not available in our budgets and the work of running the project meant that the research team is only now, at the time of writing, making full use of the data available from the project.

Fundamentally, involving research users in a purposeful and extensive way challenges the very foundations of how we are used to doing research projects. This is undoubtedly a benefit, but crucially what this means is that we have to remain flexible about the way we plan research, our projects may be uncompetitive when compared with standard research approaches received by the funding bodies, and we have to be prepared to hand over some of our autonomy as researchers.

Conclusion

There is a tendency to present user involvement as a 'good thing' but, as Beresford (2002) has pointed out, it has not only liberatory but also regressive potential. Concerns that involving users in research be successful have led to the identification of eight principles of involvement (Telford et al. 2004). Though acknowledged as having been developed with a focus on NHS research, covering 'consumers' in general, and arguably more appropriate to researcher rather than user-led research, nevertheless they offer a test of the approaches taken in the OWLV project.

We recognize that older women were not the initiators of the project (Older People's Steering Group 2004), which had 'pre-decided methods' (Thornton 2000). However, the subsequent roles of all the participants, not simply the volunteers, were agreed between the academic researchers and the older women involved in the project. The costs of involving all participants was covered, although this meant some virement within the budget, and negotiating fees for presentations once the project had ended. We have documented here some of the different skills, knowledge and experience that the volunteers brought to, as well as gained from, the project. The volunteers were involved in defining research themes and questions, undertaking life story interviews, negotiating the meanings of the findings as well as in disseminating them and generally keeping all participants informed of the progress of the research.

In these aspects, we met all but one of the principles of successful user involvement in research. Moreover, it may be argued in the OWLV project's favour that, while the methods were pre-decided, they were chosen in an attempt to address some of the limitations of mainstream theory and practice in user participation identified above. We were also able to offer perspectives on having a say from older women from different ethnic groups that are commonly lacking in work on involvement in research (cf. Telford et al. 2004).

Nevertheless, despite overcoming a number of challenges, there remained limitations to the OWLV project:

- The project failed to include hard-to-reach groups, especially housebound older women and women with dementia, communication and sensory difficulties.
- Women from such groups were not recruited partly because of the limits of our experience, speaking as the writers of this chapter, in participatory research. We had been variously involved in running discussion groups and conducting life story interviews with older women users of services, but not strictly within a framework of user involvement in research. In retrospect, we feel that with training (the eighth principle identified by Telford et al. 2004), we might have designed a project that was less ambitious in terms of the range of involvement, and been better able to anticipate and manage a number of the challenges of the project, particularly relating to the setting of ground rules for group work and the resourcing of activities.
- Arguably, the major limitation was our failure to guarantee mechanisms for taking forward the findings at the local level. One of the most important motivations for involvement for participants in the project was to carry findings into policy and practice. As one of the volunteers commented at a Toronto Group seminar presentation: 'When academics are doing things, it's just lip service . . . Most people want research and then something doing.' At the planning stage of the OWLV research, we had viewed the Sheffield BGOP pilot as providing important avenues. However, changes in the development of the initiative – especially the folding of the BGOP Network and Forum at the end of the pilot and the

refocusing of energies on the setting up of the Sheffield Congress of Elders – had a considerable impact on opportunities. Thus, we have concentrated, as have so many other projects, chiefly on reporting the way in which older women have been involved in the 'process' but not on evaluation of the end results (in terms of what the women wanted to influence, at least).

- We may have been better able to track and evaluate the impact of the OWLV initiative had we been able to achieve involvement beyond the life of the project (see section on 'Challenges to involvement' earlier in the chapter) and also if some of our contacts in different service areas who were interested in the OWLV project had not also faced the problem of having limited funds to carry forward the work with us. Thornton (2000: 16) has written that 'fatigue and disillusion can set in if involvement becomes burdensome and leads to few tangible results'. This can apply as much to the efforts of researchers and committed policy makers in promoting involvement in research as to older people taking part. It is not always easy to remain patient in tolerating the slow drip, drip impact of research that some advocates of user involvement have identified as being the most we can expect from our efforts (Osborn 1984).

Guidelines to older people's involvement in research are beginning to emerge that offer alternatives to the dominant model of involvement by public consultation used by the government, identify elements of good as well as bad practice and, most importantly, are based on the direct experiences of older people who took part. They demonstrate that developing an inclusive involvement strategy requires time, money, commitment, flexibility, confidence building and trust. However, such guidelines tend to be derived from specific initiatives (cf. Cormie and Warren 2001 for guidelines based on the Fife User Panels project but also drawing from insights from the OWLV work). The Older People's Steering Group (2004) has been looking at ideas of involvement with the aim of beginning to set some standards for national adoption. As Thornton (2000) has noted, we also need to know more about which methods older people prefer for different purposes, as well as asking why and how they may be successful in achieving results – perhaps the work of a future partnership research project.

Notes

1   Link-Age is a project set up by the Department of Work and Pensions to develop networks of services for older people. For further details, visit www.socialexclusion. gov.uk.

2   The Joseph Rowntree Foundation has been supporting a programme of research about the lives of older people since 2000. The programme was developed by and with older people themselves, working in a steering group with officers, researchers and policy advisers and has examined older people's priorities for 'living well in later life'. For full details and downloadable reports, visit the website www.jrf.org.uk.

3   Full details of INVOLVE and its activities in promoting public involvement in NHS, public health and social care research are available on its website

www.invo.org.uk. Other potential initiatives of influence include the work of the Social Exclusion Unit and the Better Services for Vulnerable People initiative.

4   The Toronto Group was set up following the Fourth International Empowerment Conference at the University of Toronto in Canada in September 1997. The group's aim is to promote and share Social Care research that empowers service users who take part in research and service users more generally. The group includes researchers, practitioners, managers, educators, service users and service user researchers. The group has run a seminar series on Research as Empowerment, funded by the Joseph Rowntree Foundation, with additional funding from INVOLVE and Race Equality Unit. For further details, contact the project co-ordinator, Rachel Purtell: r.a.purtell@ex.ac.uk.

5   In association with the Learning Media Unit (LeMU), Sheffield University (2002) *Older Women's Lives and Voices Video*, Sheffield: LeMU, University of Sheffield.

Acknowledgements

The OWLV project was funded by the Economic and Social Research Council (ESRC) Growing Older (GO) programme, award reference number L480254048 and co-directed by Lorna Warren and Tony Maltby (University of Birmingham).

As with all OWLV project publications and presentations, this chapter is dedicated to Ying Wah Cheng, who died suddenly in 2002. Ying was committed to the project and its aims, and an inspiration to us all in terms of her dedication, drive and passion for life. Special thanks also go to the volunteers and Graham McElearney, director of the video.

References

Barnes, M. (1997) *Care, Communities and Citizens*, London: Longman.
Barnes, M. (1999) 'Working with older people to evaluate the Fife User Panels Project', in M. Barnes and L. Warren (eds) *Paths to Empowerment*, Bristol: Policy Press.
Barnes, M. (2002) 'Dialogue between older people and public officials: UK experiences', in *Grey Power? Volume 1: Political Power and Influence*, Paris: Les Cahiers de la FIAPA, Action Research on Ageing (published in French and English).
Barnes, M. and Bennett-Emslie, G. (1997) *'If They Would Listen . . .' An Evaluation of the Fife User Panels*, Edinburgh: Age Concern Scotland.
Barnes, M. and Bennett, G. (1998) 'Frail bodies, courageous voices: older people influencing community care', *Health and Social Care in the Community*, 6 (2): 102–11.
Barnes, M. and Walker, A. (1996) 'Consumerism versus empowerment: a principled approach to the involvement of older service users', *Policy and Politics*, 24 (4): 375–93.
Beresford, P. (1997) 'The last social division? Revisiting the relationship between social policy, its producers and consumers', in M. May, E. Brunsdon and G. Craig (eds) *Social Policy Review 9*, London: Social Policy Association.
Beresford, P. (2002) 'User involvement in research and evaluation: liberation or regulation?', *Social Policy and Society*, 1 (2): 95–106.
Bernard, M., Phillips, J., Machin, L. and Harding Davies, V. (2000) *Women Ageing: Changing Identities, Challenging Myths*, London: Routledge.
Better Government for Older People (Programme) (1999) *Making it Happen: Report of the First Year of the Programme 1998–99*, London: Cabinet Office (available http://www.bettergovernmentforolderpeople.gov.uk) (accessed 9 April 2000).
Better Government for Older People (BGOP) (Advisory Group) (2000a) *Our Present for the Future*, Wolverhampton: BGOP.

Better Government for Older People (BGOP) (Steering Committee) (2000b) *All Our Futures: The Report of the Better Government for Older People Steering Committee*, Wolverhampton: BGOP.

Boaz, A. and Hayden, C. (2000) *Listening to Local Older People: Progress on Consultation in the 28 Better Government for Older People Pilots*, Warwick: Local Government Centre, University of Warwick.

Booth, T. and Booth, W. (1996) 'Sounds of silence: narrative research with inarticulate subjects', *Disability and Society*, 11 (1): 55–69.

Booth, T. and Booth, W. (1998) *Growing Up with Parents who have Learning Difficulties*, London: Routledge.

Bornat, J. (1993) 'Life experience', in M. Bernard and K. Meade (eds) *Women Come of Age*, London: Edward Arnold.

Bowes, A. (1996) 'Evaluating an empowering research strategy: reflections on action-research with South Asian women', *Sociological Research Online*, 1 (1) (available http://www.socres online.org.uk/socresonline/1/1/1.html) (accessed 2 July 1999).

Burgess, R. (1984) 'The unstructured interview as a conversation', in R. Burgess (ed.) *Field Research: Sourcebook and Field Manual*, Hemel Hempstead: George Allen and Unwin.

Butt, J. and Mirza, K. (1996) *Social Care and Black Communities*, London: HMSO.

Cabinet Office (1999) *Modernising Government*, London: Cabinet Office.

Carter, T. and Beresford, P. (2000) *Age and Change: Models of Involvement for Older People*, York: Joseph Rowntree Foundation by York Publishing Services.

Centre for Social Action (1999) *About the Centre*, Leicester: Centre for Social Action, De Montfort University.

Cook, J., Maltby, T. and Warren, L. (2004) 'A participatory approach to older women's quality of life', in A. Walker and C. Hagan Hennessey (eds) *Growing Older: Quality of Life in Old Age*, Buckingham: Open University Press.

Cormie, J. and Warren, L. (2001) *Working with Older People: Guidelines for Running Discussion Groups and Influencing Practice*, Bristol: Policy Press.

Cornwell, J. (1984) *Hard-earned Lives: Accounts of Health and Illness from East London*, London: Tavistock.

Counsel and Care (eds) (1994) *More Power to our Elders: Promoting Empowerment for Older People*, London: Counsel and Care.

Curtis, Z. (1993) 'On being a woman in the pensioners' movement', in J. Johnson and R. Slater (eds) *Ageing and Later Life*, London: Sage.

Curtis, Z. (1995) 'Gaining confidence – speaking out', in R. Jack (ed.) *Empowerment in Community Care*, London: Chapman and Hall.

Department of Health (1991) *Managers and Practitioners: Guide to Care Management and Assessment*, London: HMSO.

Department of Health (1997) *The New NHS: Modern and Dependable*, London: DoH.

Department of Health (1998) *Modernising Social Services: Promoting Independence, Improving Protection, Reviewing Standards*, Cm 4169, London: The Stationery Office.

Department of Health (1999) *Patient and Public Involvement in the New NHS*, London: DoH.

Department of Health (2000) *Research and Development for a First Class Service*, London: DoH.

Department of Social Security (for the Ministerial Group on Older People) (1998) *Building a Better Britain for Older People*, Hayes, Middlesex: Welfare Reform.

Dingwall, R. (1980) 'Ethics and ethnography', *Sociological Review*, 28 (4): 871–91.

Fisk, M. (1997) 'Older people as researchers', in R. Sykes (ed.) *Putting Older People in the Picture: Conference Report*, Oxford: Anchor Trust.

Gearing, B. and Dant, T. (1990) 'Doing biographical research', in S. Peace (ed.) *Researching Social Gerontology: Concepts, Methods and Issues*, London: Sage.

Hanley, B., Bradburn, J., Barnes, M., Evans, C., Goodare, H., Kelson, M., Kent, A., Oliver, S., Thomas, S. and Wallcraft, J. (2003) *Involving the Public in NHS, Public Health, and Social Care Research: Briefing Notes for Researchers*, 2nd edn, Eastleigh, Hampshire: INVOLVE.

Hayden, C. and Boaz, A. (2000) *Making a Difference: Evaluation Report*, Wolverhampton: BGOP.

Hazan, H. (1994) *Old Age: Constructions and Deconstructions*, Cambridge: Cambridge University Press.

Hobman, D. (1994) 'What price consumer choice', in Counsel and Care (eds), *More Power to Our Elders: Promoting Empowerment for Older People*, London: Counsel and Care.

hooks, b. (1986) 'Sisterhood: political solidarity between women', *Feminist Review*, 23: 125–38.

Kelly, C. and Breinlinger, S. (1995) 'Identity and injustice: exploring women's participation in collective action', *Journal of Community and Applied Social Psychology*, 5: 41–57.

Kemshall, H. and Littlechild, R. (eds) (2000) *User Involvement and Participation in Social Care: Research Informing Practice*, London: Jessica Kingsley.

Lockey, R., Sitzia, J., Gillingham, T., Millyard, J., Miller, C., Ahmed, S., Beales, A., Bennett, C., Parfoot, S., Sigrist, J. and Worthing and Southlands Hospitals NHS Trust (2004) *Report Summary: Training for Service User Involvement in Health and Social Care Research – A Study of Training Provision and Participants' Experiences*, Eastleigh, Hampshire: INVOLVE.

National Health Service Executive, Institute of Health Service Management and The National Health Service Confederation (1998) *In the Public Interest: Developing a Strategy for Public Participation in the NHS*, London: DoH.

Newman, J. (2001) *Modernising Governance: New Labour, Policy and Society*, London: Sage.

Nolan, M. (2000) 'Towards person-centred care for older people', in A. Warnes, L. Warren and M. Nolan (eds) *Care Services for Later Life*, London: Jessica Kingsley.

Older People's Steering Group (2004) *Older People Shaping Policy and Practice*, York: Joseph Rowntree Foundation.

Osborn, A. (1984) 'Research utilisation: another Cinderella?', in D. B. Bromley (ed.) *Gerontology: Social and Behavioural Perspectives*, London: Croom Helm.

Patel, N. (1993) 'Healthy margins: black elders' care – models, policies and prospects', in W. Ahmad (ed.) *'Race' and Health in Contemporary Britain*, Buckingham: Open University Press.

Peace, S. (ed.) (1999) *Involving Older People in Research: 'An Amateur Doing the Work of a Professional'*, London: Centre for Policy on Ageing.

Plummer, K. (1990) 'Herbert Blumer and the life history tradition', *Symbolic Interaction*, 13 (2): 125–44.

Rappert, B. (1997) 'Users and social science research: policy, problems and possibilities', *Sociological Research Online*, 2: 3 (available http://www.socresonline.org.uk/socresonline/2//3/3.html) (accessed 7 April 2000).

Reinharz, S. (1992) *Feminist Methods in Social Research*, Oxford: Oxford University Press.

Richards, S. (1994) 'Enabling research: elderly people', *Research, Policy and Planning*, 12 (2): 5–6.

Royle, J., Steel, R., Hanley, B. and Bradburn, J. (2001) *Getting Involved in Research: A Guide for Consumers*, Winchester: Consumers in NHS Research Support Unit.

Ruth, J-E. and Kenyon, G. (1996) 'Introduction', *Ageing and Society*, 16 (6): 653–8.

Sharpe, P. A. (1995) 'Older women and health services: moving from ageism to empowerment', *Women and Health*, 22 (3): 9–23.

Simney, M. (1998) 'The politics of ageing', in M. Bernard and J. Phillips (eds) *The Social Policy of Old Age: Moving into the 21st Century*, London: Centre for Policy on Ageing.

Stevenson, O. and Parsloe, P. (1993) *Community Care and Empowerment*, York: Joseph Rowntree Foundation.

Telford, R., Boote, J. and Cooper, C. (2004) 'What does it mean to involve consumers successfully in NHS research? A consensus study', *Health Expectations*, 7: 209–20.

Thornton, P. (2000) *Older People Speaking Out: Developing Opportunities for Influence*, York: Joseph Rowntree Foundation by York Publishing Services.

Thornton, P. and Tozer, R. (1994) *Involving Older People in Planning and Evaluating Community Care: A Review of Initiatives*, York: Social Policy Research Unit, University of York.

Thornton, P. and Tozer, R. (1995) *Having a Say in Change: Older People and Community Care*, York: Joseph Rowntree Foundation.

Tozer, R. and Thornton, P. (1995) *A Meeting of Minds: Older People as Research Advisers*, York: Social Policy Research Unit, University of York.

Walker, A. (1998) 'Speaking for themselves: the new politics of old age in Europe', *Education and Ageing*, 13 (1): 13–36.

Walker, A. and Maltby, T. (1997) *Ageing Europe*, Buckingham: Open University Press.

Warren, L. (1999) 'Empowerment: the path to partnership?', in M. Barnes and L. Warren (eds) *Paths to Empowerment*, Bristol: Policy Press.

Warren, L. and Maltby, T. (2000) 'Averil Osborn and participatory research: involving older people in change', in A. Warnes, L. Warren and M. Nolan (eds) *Care Services for Later Life*, London: Jessica Kingsley Publishers.

Warren, L., Cook, J., Clarke, N., Hadfield, P., Haywood-Reed, P., Millen, L., Parkinson, M., Robinson, J. and Winfield, W. (2003) 'Working with older women in research: some methods-based issues, *Quality in Ageing*, 4 (4): 24–31.

Williams, M. (2004) 'Discursive democracy and New Labour: five ways in which decision makers manage citizens agendas in public participation initiatives', *Sociological Research Online*, 9 (3), (available http://www.socresonline.org.uk/9/3/williams.html) (accessed 31 August 2004).

Wray, S. (2003) 'Women growing older: agency, ethnicity and culture', *Sociology* 37 (3): 511–27.

Chapter 17

Service user involvement at all stages of the research process

Matthew Harris

Introduction

Service user involvement in planning and delivery of care is not a new concept. There has long been a tradition within the voluntary sector of organizing and delivering services around the priorities and needs of users, to support mainstream health and social services (Truman and Raine 2002). In recent years, user participation in the planning and development of health care has become central to government policy. Patients now have a significant role in determining and shaping services, identifying their own health needs and making choices about their own health care (Department of Health 2000, 2001; Trivedi and Wykes 2002; Rutter et al. 2004).

If service users' needs are to be key components to improving service delivery, then their views should be central to the evaluation of service provision. However, the extent to which this is carried out in practice and the methods typically used are still at a rudimentary stage (Truman and Raine 2002). Entwistle et al. (1998) suggested that involving users in research design can help improve the quality of health research, as the lay perspective provides insight into areas that may be overlooked by professionals, yet cause significant problems for patients and carers. Not only should health research be valid science, but also it should be deemed to be valuable by those who live with the medical condition or use the services of interest.

This chapter focuses on the potential for service user involvement at each stage of the research cycle, from initial planning and research design to dissemination. It draws on experiences gained from a European Commission funded project (InfoPark), which aimed to investigate the perceptions of older people with Parkinson's disease and their carers about information provision. We wanted to evaluate patients' and carers' experiences, views and opinions about their needs and use the findings as the basis for developing more appropriate user-focused information materials. The central role of service users in the development and execution of the research project ensured that the most relevant issues were investigated, appropriate conclusions were drawn and the results were effectively implemented.

Background to InfoPark

The 'InfoPark' project (http://infopark.uwcm.ac.uk) is a European collaborative research study focusing on the information needs of older people affected by Parkinson's disease. A fundamental principle of the research team was that, particularly in chronic conditions such as Parkinson's disease, patients and carers are often the 'experts', yet their perspectives on their needs and experiences of disease management are rarely heard. By making patients and carers an integral part of the research team, InfoPark aimed to identify and address their real information needs and narrow the gap between users' and professionals' perceptions of good practice in information giving and clinical decision making.

Although the project focused on Parkinson's disease, the project aimed to identify and explore issues that were of relevance to older people with chronic conditions in general. Certainly all chronic illnesses typically cause physical and psychological difficulties, socio-economic problems and social isolation that can have an enduring negative impact upon the individual patient's and their family's quality of life. Some are severely and chronically restricted in performing basic activities of daily living and heavily dependent on others for help with most aspects of everyday life. Others experience less severe disability, with intermittent episodes of ill health, of varying intensity and duration. All not only have specific information needs concerning their condition, but also have a core of common requirements (Department of Health 2001). Unfortunately, these needs often go unmet.

The concept of user empowerment, as it relates to health care, implies that patient and carer autonomy may be optimized through the provision of care that assists them to assert control over their lives (Faulkner 2001). Empowerment can be achieved through the provision of information and recognition of the patients' right to be involved in decisions concerning their own treatment. Encouraging an equal role in decision making by involving patients, carers and professionals as partners in care is increasingly promoted as the best model of health care provision (Charles et al. 1997; Holman and Lorig 2000). However, both the perceived resistance of health professionals to patient and carer empowerment and traditional paternalistic patient–doctor relationships appear still to act as barriers to involvement for many individuals (Evans et al. 2003).

With the growing emphasis of user involvement within research, 'InfoPark' brings together a range of academics, clinicians and user organizations from seven European countries. The research team in each country was planned to include both users and professionals and three of the national research teams are led by user organizations: Associacion Parkinson Madrid (Spain), Tartu Parkinson's Disease Society (Estonia) and Associacao Portuguesa de deontes de Parkinson (Portugal). The eighth research partner is the European Parkinson's Disease Association (EPDA) that helps to promote a Europe-wide perspective and effective dissemination of the project findings.

The aim was to have patients and carers and their representatives as central partners and to act as key decision makers at all stages of the research process. This involved users' identifying and prioritizing topics of interest, commissioning, designing and managing the research, collecting, analysing and interpreting data, disseminating results and lastly evaluating the outcomes. To explore comprehensively the key issues relevant to improving information needs, it was pivotal for researchers and users to draw upon each other's respective knowledge and insights. Although users may not be experts in scientific methodology or design, they may address issues central to users' concerns, irrespective of their research knowledge (Barnard 1998).

Identifying project objectives

By making patients and carers an integral part of the research team, InfoPark aimed to identify and address their real information needs and narrow the gap between users' and professionals' perceptions of good practice in information giving and clinical decision making. Patient organizations and individual consumers had been involved with discussions about the project objectives from an early stage and ensured that the final research protocol was practical and user focused. This is likely to have contributed to the success of the application for research funding (against strong competition), as it later emerged that consumers were themselves involved in influencing the research agenda and played a prominent role in the peer review process.

Our review of the available literature and consultations with a wide range of professionals, together with our own personal experiences and views, formed the basis of the initial research protocol. This was then discussed with service users. They identified some additional areas that they considered to be important and that needed to be addressed (for example, the role of complementary therapies, sexual issues and safety to travel) and placed a different emphasis on other issues (for example they prioritized information on prognosis, non-drug management and emotional issues and were less concerned about pathological mechanisms and causes of the illness and reasons for choice of medication).

From all the preliminary investigations, four key areas were identified that addressed all the issues that had been highlighted:

- Participants' knowledge prior to diagnosis: their experiences of the illness; who was approached about the illness and why.
- The information given at the time of diagnosis: satisfaction with the information received; additional information required; from whom the information was received; any problems experienced at that time.
- The information received post-diagnosis: the types of information they needed; the types of information received; the topics of information received and needed, including medical and non-medical management, coping with daily living, social issues and emotional needs.
- What information participants thought should be available: which information was most beneficial; the form in which it should be presented; who should be responsible for providing information.

These were the issues that formed the basis of the subsequent empirical research.

Choosing the methodology

Many problems arising in research can be attributed to a failure to recognize the purpose to which each available methodology is best suited (Winter 2000; Edwards and Staniszewska 2000). All research depends on collecting particular sorts of evidence through specific methods, for a specific purpose and each methodology has strengths and weaknesses (Mays and Pope 1995). By systematically determining which is the most appropriate approach in a particular situation, it is hoped to maximize the strengths and minimize the weaknesses of the study.

The InfoPark project used qualitative methodology, and specifically semistructured interviews, to explore the information needs of older people with Parkinson's disease and their lay carers. It was considered that this method would allow the central focus to be placed on individual needs and opinions and exploration of personal experiences. The interview schedule was constructed around the four key areas of interest that had been identified in the preliminary studies. Open questions and prompts were used to encourage participants to talk about their own experiences. The aim was for them to discuss issues in their own words, while providing some structure to the interview and ensuring that all the areas of interest were covered. There was also the flexibility for additional questions to be asked and to allow patients and carers the opportunity to raise issues they felt were important, thus ensuring they were active participants in the research process.

The importance of rigour when using qualitative methods is no less than with quantitative investigations. It was necessary to provide a lot of training and supervision to those partners from user organizations without prior experience of undertaking qualitative research. The importance of the researchers remaining neutral and not introducing bias into the process of data collection (or later analysis) was constantly emphasized and quality assurance systems were put into place. Training workshops were conducted to ensure that research standards were consistently high. This inevitably added to the time taken to complete the work and to the financial costs. Service users were unused to the discipline of following research protocols, meeting deadlines, working within the constraints of research budgets and effective project management was all important.

Conducting the empirical research

The need for independent ethical approval for all health and social care related research (including research that is non-invasive and studies using 'healthy volunteer subjects') is now widely accepted and a prerequisite for undertaking data collection in most countries. The importance of gaining fully informed consent from all participants requires researchers to ensure that they give a clear and balanced account of what the research aims to achieve, why the subject has been asked to participate, an outline of the methods, possible benefits and risks, legal rights and safeguards (including the opportunity to withdraw at any time), and how information collected will be used (Consumers for Ethics in Research (CERES) 2003). Issues that are not considered important by researchers, and so not discussed, may be a source of major concern to potential participants and impact on recruitment. The involvement of patient organizations and individual consumers in helping to refine study consent procedures and improving content and phrasing of study information leaflets ensures that the research can be explained to potential volunteers most effectively (Koops and Lindley 2002).

In the InfoPark study, purposive sampling was used to identify suitable people to interview. This is a deliberately non-random method of sampling, which enabled researchers to focus on a pre-selected group of interviewees most likely to provide in-depth information of the population of interest (Silverman 2000). We wished to target people aged 65 years and over and who had been clinically diagnosed with Parkinson's disease, but otherwise represented a broad range of impairment and handicap, were from different socio-economic backgrounds, and received varied support from informal and formal caregivers. We hoped this would help to ensure that we obtained representative views of the whole population, rather than recruitment of disproportionate numbers of the more able and articulate who were most easily identified and most likely to participate.

The active involvement of user organizations gave us access to a large pool of subjects and we were able to target individuals with particular characteristics. Regular updates about progress of the research were reported in Parkinson's Association magazines and newsletters and individual participants were able to keep abreast of the findings and conclusions of the study. This helped to give a sense of ownership and active participation in the research process and ensured that we were able to recruit a large number of suitable research subjects within a short time period.

Individuals working with user organizations were involved not only with planning and advising about the content of the research interviews and recruiting potential participants, but also with data collection itself. Training workshops were organized to ensure the reliability and validity of the conduct of the interviews, with the more experienced researchers from academic backgrounds teaching their colleagues about the theory and practice of data collection. The importance of making best use of the limited time available for interview and the need to ensure objectivity and avoidance of bias were of special concern. At the suggestion of some service users, interviews were arranged with participants at times that coincided as far as possible with their medication and 'on-time', so that discussion was facilitated and best use was made of the available time. Specific areas of interest were introduced to participants with questions printed in a large font size so that they were easily visible and understood. At the end of the formal interview, participants were asked to inform their friends with Parkinson's disease of our research and to encourage them to contact us if they were interested in taking part. Thus, interviewees themselves became part of the project team.

Analysing the data

Analysis drew on grounded theory procedures and used the method of constant comparison (Glaser and Strauss 1967). Data collection and data analysis continued concurrently. This iterative process enabled project partners to pursue emerging themes in subsequent interviews and search for deviant/negative cases. By analysing the data concurrently, interviews continued until no new information was generated (i.e. data saturation was achieved). To ensure accuracy and detail of information, all interviews were tape-recorded using a high quality tape recorder. Verbatim transcriptions of the recorded data were conducted as soon as possible after the interview to aid memory of circumstances and characteristics of individual participants. Detailed field notes taken during the interviews aided this process. All transcripts were anonymized and all participants were promised confidentiality, with letters and numbers substituted for participants' names. The transcripts were checked to ensure accuracy and, to permit familiarity, the data transcripts were read repeatedly.

After transcription, word transcripts were transferred into a qualitative analysis software package (HyperResearch) for coding. The transcripts were coded independently and a 'coding template' was developed. The initial codes were largely descriptive and allowed for variation within each category. Analysis involved three processes that overlapped; open coding, where data were broken open to identify relevant categories, axial coding, where categories were refined, developed and relationships identified and lastly selective coding where 'core categories' were developed linking all other categories and sub categories in the study together. The coding template continued to evolve as new information was collected. Once coding had been completed, all the information was transferred back to a Word processing package for further in-depth analysis.

All transcripts were coded by project partners. In addition, interview transcripts were coded by a second colleague to minimize bias. Samples were compared by checking the codes assigned to segments of text in the transcripts line by line. The codes that were very similar, sometimes using identical terms or forms of words, were discussed and agreed to mean the same thing. The comparison of agreement between codes confirmed a good level of reproducibility. Each interview was then written into a descriptive account to explore similarities and differences for each theme between the participants. This involved analysing codes within participants' transcripts and looking for any comparative or contrasting views. These accounts were collated to produce the final analysis, which illustrated both common and 'negative' themes.

Development of information materials and dissemination

From the results of the empirical research members of the InfoPark team identified key topics to form the basis of information materials for patients, carers and professionals. Group workshops and individual discussions were held to allow everyone to contribute and refine the content and design of the information material. These followed recognized guidelines, aiming to be concise, with a structured design and appropriate illustration. Opinions of service users were highly influential in the design and layout of the information material. Users were able to provide knowledge and expertise concerning strengths and weaknesses of past and present information material and advised on a number of issues such as layout (simple and consistent), font size (large), colour (limited), language (non-technical, non-patronizing and non-alarmist) and most importantly content.

The final version of the materials grouped topics under the broad headings of:

- Learning about your illness, what carers need to know (symptoms, causes, how the diagnosis is made, treatments and therapies).
- Getting on with life (keeping active, looking to the future, dealing with stress and emotions, sleep, problems with thinking, financial and legal issues).
- Asking the right questions to the right people (frequently asked questions and who best to ask).
- Where to get more information (useful contacts and organizations, written materials and websites).
- Issues of relevance to carers include information on basic caring skills, helping with lifting and moving, practical aids and adaptations, managing stress, carers' rights and being more assertive, accepting help and respite breaks.

- Information for professionals includes working in partnership with patients and carers, sharing information and confidentiality, being sensitive to patient and carer wishes, the Team Approach to management, telling the diagnosis and improving verbal and written communications with patients and their families.

Altogether 42 'infosheets' were developed, each addressing a particular topic. Information materials were developed with the notion that patients, carers and professionals can select infosheets that are of personal interest at any particular time and relevant to their specific needs. Drafts were developed in English, piloted with experts and users in the United Kingdom and modified in the light of their comments. A glossary of terms and suggestions for sources of further information were added. Final versions were translated, with appropriate national and cultural modifications and available in traditional paper copy, electronic format and on the Internet. Following comments from service users, the website was designed with simpler navigation and larger buttons.

Expert round table discussions

To monitor the project's progress, expert round table discussions were held at several stages of the research process, from inception to completion. Those attending the round table discussions were European 'expert' patients and carers and their representatives, who were not directly involved in the research project, but with personal experience and knowledge of living with a chronic disabling condition. The round table discussions served as a means of identifying appropriate research questions, exploring practical issues associated with the methodologies, interpretation of the project's findings and initial dissemination of the project outcomes. They provided also an opportunity to explore the relevance of the results to other chronic conditions and for the researchers to develop further ideas in collaboration with user organizations, individual patients, carers and health professionals.

Three expert round table discussions were conducted at stages throughout the project. The first of the expert round table discussions involved asking individuals to provide initial views and opinions concerning what issues would be most appropriate to explore with patients, carers and professionals regarding information needs. These, together with the results of the literature search and project workshop discussions, shaped the content of the interview schedule.

A second expert round table discussion explored the empirical results of the project and their relevance to older people with chronic illness across Europe. The aim of the meeting was to present the findings to a wider audience so that areas of agreement, consensus or variance could be identified. By consulting a second group of experts the InfoPark collaboration wanted to identify if the information needs of patients with Parkinson's disease and their lay carers were similar or dissimilar to other chronic conditions. The outcome contributed directly to the development and structure of the information materials.

A final expert round table discussion was conducted to identify best practice, test validity of findings across a range of disabilities and improve dissemination. The aim was to establish if the information material designed by the collaboration could provide a basic template for information material focusing on other chronic conditions. The research process is summarized in Figure 17.1.

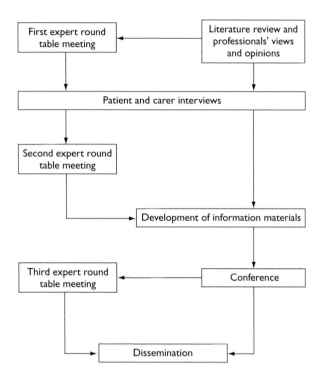

Figure 17.1 The research process.

Conclusion

Conducting research is a very rigorous and time-consuming process. Involving users in planning and conducting research presents an extra challenge for researchers, but is more than justified by the potential benefits. For service users' participation to be productive, researchers must believe that the value and validity of their work will be enhanced. There needs to be a strategy for involving users more effectively in all aspects of research, from planning, commissioning and data collection and analysis, through to the dissemination and presentation of the findings (Barnard 1998; Donovan et al. 2002; Trivedi and Wykes 2002). Certainly, our experience from the InfoPark project is that the benefits of such an approach can far outweigh any burden.

Acknowledgements

This chapter was written on behalf of the InfoPark Collaboration, funded by the European Commission under the Fifth Framework Quality of Life Programme, Contract no. PLK6 2000-00303.

References

Barnard, S. (1998) 'Consumer involvement and inter-agency collaboration in clinical audit', *Health and Social Care in the Community*, 6: 130–42.

Charles, C., Gafne, A. and Whelan, T. (1997) 'Shared decision making in the medical encounter: what does it mean (or it takes at least two to tango)', *Social Science and Medicine*, 44: 681–92.

Consumers for Ethics in Research (CERES) (2003) *Health Research and You*, London: CERES.

Department of Health (2000) *The NHS Plan: A Plan for Investment a Plan for Reform*, London: DoH.

Department of Health (2001) *The Expert Patient: A New Approach to Chronic Disease Management for the 21st Century*, London: DoH.

Donovan, J., Mill, N., Smith, M., Brindle, L., Jacoby, A., Peters, T., Frankel, S., Neal, D., Hamdy, F. and Little, P. (2002) 'Improving design and conduct of randomised trails by embedding them in qualitative research: ProtecT (prostate testing for cancer and treatment) study', *British Medical Journal*, 325: 766–9.

Edwards, C. and Staniszewska, S. (2000) 'Accessing the user's perspective', *Health and Social Care in the Community*, 8: 417–24.

Entwistle, V., Renfrew, M., Yearly, S., Forrester, J. and Lamont, T. (1998) 'Lay perspectives: advantages for health research', *British Medical Journal*, 316: 463–6.

Evans, S., Tritter, J., Barley, V., Daykin, N., McNeill, J., Palmer, N., Rimmer, J., Sanidas, M. and Turton, P. (2003) 'User involvement in UK cancer services: bridging the policy gap', *European Journal of Cancer Care*, 12: 331–8.

Faulkner, M. (2001) 'Empowerment, disempowerment and the care of older people', *Nursing Older People*, 13: 18–20.

Glaser, B. and Strauss, A. (1967) *The Discovery of Grounded Theory*, Chicago: Aldine.

Holman, H. and Lorig, K. (2000) 'Patients as partners in managing chronic disease', *British Medical Journal*, 320: 526–7.

Koops, L. and Lindley, R. (2002) 'Thrombolysis for acute ischaemic stroke: consumer involvement in design of new randomised controlled trails', *British Medical Journal*, 325: 415–7.

Mays, N. and Pope, C. (1995) 'Qualitative research: rigour and qualitative research', *British Medical Journal*, 311: 109–12.

Rutter, D., Manley, C., Weaver, T., Crawford, M. and Fulop, N. (2004) 'Patients or partners? Case studies of user involvement in the planning and delivery of adult mental health services in London', *Social Science and Medicine*, 58: 1973–84.

Silverman, D. (2000) *Doing Qualitative Research: A Practical Handbook*, London: Sage.

Trivedi, P. and Wykes, T. (2002) 'From passive subjects to equal partners', *British Journal of Psychiatry*, 181: 468–72.

Truman, C. and Raine, P. (2002) 'Experience and meaning of user involvement: some explorations from a community mental health project', *Health and Social Care in the Community*, 10: 136–43.

Winter, G. (2000) *A Comparative Discussion of the Notion of 'Validity' in Qualitative and Quantitative Research* (available http://www.nova.edu/ssss/QR/QR4–3/winter.html) (accessed 11 April 2003).

Chapter 18

Working together to undertake research

Ruth Northway and Paul Wheeler

Introduction

This chapter focuses on one research study undertaken during the period 1999–2000. The study brought together a mental health service user group (ForUs) and a group of university-based lecturers in a project to explore the views of mental health service users concerning their experience of medication and other therapies. The chapter is written by the lecturer responsible for co-ordinating the project (Ruth) and someone who, at the time of the study, was one of the student nurses involved in data collection (Paul).

Accounts of collaborative and participative research have been criticized for failing to provide readers with sufficient information concerning the process of such research (Reason 1998), which limits the extent to which researchers can learn from the experience of others. The chapter will, therefore, concentrate primarily upon the conduct of the study rather than on the findings, and personal reflections will be included where appropriate.

Background to study

In 1999, ForUs contacted the School of Care Sciences at the University of Glamorgan with a view to undertaking a research study on their behalf. As a group, they had identified concerns regarding the medications prescribed for mental health problems, their effects, the information provided for service users concerning medication, and the accessibility of other therapies. They had previously undertaken a small pilot study but, while local service providers had been receptive to this study, it became apparent that it was also seen as lacking 'academic rigour' and, because of this, there was a danger that it could be ignored (Parker and Northway 2002). It had thus been agreed that the support of an academic department would be helpful.

The School of Care Sciences agreed to provide the assistance requested. Financial resources to undertake the study were limited but it was agreed that data collection could be undertaken by appropriately trained student nurses thus reducing costs while at the same time providing a useful learning opportunity for those students. One of the authors (Ruth) was asked to take on responsibility for co-ordination of the project in June 1999.

The first challenge to be addressed was to develop a method of working that would ensure the rigour of the study while also ensuring that ForUs retained ownership of the study, its focus, and the research process. Ruth initially met with members of the ForUs Committee to explore further the background to the study, their concerns regarding medication and other therapies, and their wishes concerning the research. The need to take a balanced approach to data collection in order to prevent any bias was also discussed.

Acceptable methods of managing the project were also explored. It was agreed that a project steering group would be established but members of the ForUs Committee felt that they did not all wish to be directly involved in this. Instead it was decided that one member of the committee, who had an interest in research, would become a member of the project steering group and that he would liaise between the two groups. It was further agreed that minutes of all project steering group meetings would be forwarded to the ForUs Committee and that no key decisions regarding the research would be taken without their prior approval.

It was agreed that the aims of the project were:

- to determine the views of users of outpatient facilities, day hospitals and day centres regarding the medication and other treatments that they receive
- to undertake research that would be informed at all stages by the perspective of mental health service users
- to inform local policy and practice.

Reflections of the project co-ordinator

I came to this project with some experience of undertaking a participatory research study (Northway 1998). I was thus committed to the development of strategies that would promote the participation of people who use health and social care services in all stages of the research process. However, my previous study had, in comparison, been a much smaller scale project. The thought of taking on the management of this study was a little daunting in that it was a study commissioned by service users themselves. Lines and levels of accountability thus needed to be clearly established and maintained. In addition, it was a study that would involve data collection in a variety of settings, and in which student nurses would be involved as data collectors. Therefore, I had accountability not only as a researcher but also as a nurse and as a lecturer. Nonetheless, not being one to be put off by a challenge, it was also an exciting opportunity for me to try to put into practice my commitment to user involvement in research.

Preparation for study

In preparation for the study, the project steering group was established and, as agreed, involved a representative of ForUs. This group met regularly throughout the project. It was agreed that the most appropriate method of data collection was a structured interview since this would overcome any difficulties that participants might have with self-completion of questionnaires while also providing the opportunity for clarification of any questions should the need arise. In developing the interview schedule, the starting point was the concerns expressed by ForUs. It was important, however, to ensure that any issues in the wider literature relating to medication and other therapies were also considered and included where appropriate. A literature search was thus undertaken in relation to the effects of medication, compliance and non-compliance, information giving, others forms of treatment and support and the views of service users (see Northway et al. 2001a). This literature review was also shared with members of ForUs so that their study could be placed in the context of other relevant work. The resulting interview schedule was piloted with members of ForUs, amended, and then their approval sought before finalizing the tool.

Careful negotiation had to be undertaken with research sites in order to secure access for fieldwork. What was encouraging, however, was that all settings welcomed the research and that, in some, managers expressed a view that it would be good for their staff to be involved as data collectors in similar research since it would provide an ideal opportunity to listen to the views of people who use services.

Since data collection would be undertaken in a range of health and social services settings it was necessary to seek and obtain the approval of both the local research scrutiny committee and the local research ethics committee. The former assessed the scientific merit of the study while the latter scrutinized the ethical issues. Ethical issues in this study arose for a number of reasons. First, there was the fact that users of mental health services would be deemed to be 'vulnerable' subjects and, therefore, matters relating to informed consent and ensuring voluntary participation needed to be carefully considered and appropriate strategies put in place. The second area that needed to be carefully addressed was the use of student nurses as data collectors. Careful attention had to be paid to how students would be both trained and supported. Third year students undertaking the learning disability and mental health branches were invited to become data collectors. Thirteen volunteered and were trained.

Reflections of a student nurse

As a student undertaking a BSc in learning disability nursing following the project 2000 syllabus, I, like fellow members of my cohort, had undertaken a research module in the early part of my training. This covered such subjects as the difference between qualitative and quantitative research, the research process and how to critique research. As part of the assessment of the module, we were required to critique a piece of research. This provided us with practical experience of critiquing. Additionally, to satisfy the honours component of the degree, we were aware that we were required to undertake a dissertation, which necessitated us completing a literature review on our chosen subject. However, the syllabus did not provide for us to undertake research ourselves as part of our training. The corollary of this was that although we had a theoretical knowledge of the research process and its relevance to nursing, we had minimal practical experience of this process.

The opportunity to act as interviewers on a research project was, therefore, an unexpected opportunity to be able to gain experience of interviewing that would otherwise have been denied us.

It was agreed that each student would spend one week working as a data collector in one service setting and that their time there would be considered to be a clinical placement since it would provide the opportunity for the development of clinical as well as research skills. It was also agreed that a minimum of two students would be assigned to each setting to provide peer support. Having recruited students, it was then necessary that training was provided. It was also felt essential that the user involvement dimension was reflected in this training. The representative of ForUs involved in the project steering group was therefore involved in the training day provided for the students.

Reflections of a student nurse

> Having volunteered for the research, we were provided with a day of training that gave us insight into the background to the project, namely that the research had been commissioned by a service user group. It also provided us with the opportunity to practice using the interview schedule in a 'safe' environment. Additional topics that were covered included confidentiality, data collection and handling, ethical issues of pertinence to the project and informed consent. The information conveyed to us during the training session was also provided in the form of a handbook that we were able to take with us for future reference.

As the above reflection details, a handbook was provided for all students so that this could act as a resource while they were out 'in the field'. In addition, two other forms of support were provided. First, there was a designated 'on call' lecturer for each day of data collection and their details were provided for both the students and the managers of the data collection sites. Second, students were required to return data to the designated lecturer at the university at the end of each day. This then provided the opportunity for debriefing if required.

Undertaking the study

Preparation for the study was perhaps a more complex process than actually undertaking the research. It was also the stage at which ForUs had the least involvement except via regular updates of progress in project steering group meetings.

Some logistical difficulties were experienced such as cancellation of outpatient clinics and fewer clients than expected using 'drop in' facilities on certain days. In such instances, it was necessary to make some adjustments to the timing of fieldwork and, in one instance, to return to a site for a further week. Throughout this period some students did make use of the 'on call' lecturer. This was mainly in relation to the logistical difficulties detailed above. What was encouraging, however, was that some of the students had thought of strategies for overcoming difficulties before contacting the lecturer. They sought contact to discuss their suggestions and to seek approval for suggested courses of action.

A further aspect of user involvement at this stage was the involvement of mental health service users as participants in the study. As the reflection below indicates, some insights were gained from this aspect of the process that might assist in future studies.

Reflections of the project co-ordinator

> On one occasion, I was the designated lecturer on call when a message was received early in the morning from one of the student nurses saying that they were unable to undertake the data collection that day due to illness. Not having time to contact another student nurse and ask them if they could stand in, I decided that I would undertake the data collection myself. This meant spending the day with another of the students in a social services 'drop in' day centre. A number of those attending were willing to participate following explanation of what the study was about. However, others indicated that they had taken part in research before but that nothing had changed in their lives as a result of such research. They were, therefore, unwilling to participate in the current study. This reinforced the need to ensure that findings of research are fed back to those who take part and that findings are utilized to inform service development.

Records were kept of the number of people approached regarding participation and the number agreeing to take part. In total, 99 people took part giving an overall response rate of 55.6 per cent. Of these, 49 were men and 50 were women.

Findings and recommendations

Data analysis was primarily undertaken by the research team. However, emerging results were discussed in project steering group meetings and thus were fed back to ForUs at regular intervals. As was noted in the introduction, the focus of this chapter is primarily upon the process of research rather than upon the findings. However, some key findings are worthy of note (see Northway et al. 2001a).

Most respondents were currently taking medication for mental health problems or had taken such medication in the previous five years. Both positive and negative experiences of taking such medication had been experienced. However, only 47 people reported that they had been given verbal information concerning their medication, 5 that they had been given only written information and 13 that they had been given both written and verbal. When asked how they would prefer information to be given, 47 people indicated that their preference was for both written and verbal information; 51 people indicated that their medication had been reviewed in the past 6 months, and a further 12, that a review had taken place between 6 and 12 months ago. However, some variations between service settings were apparent. Participants reported being offered a range of therapies other than medication the most common being art and craft work (70 people).

The following recommendations were made based on the findings:

- that current areas of good practice be maintained and built upon to ensure that such practice is universal
- that work be undertaken to ensure that timely, appropriate, and understandable information is provided for people who use mental health services
- that apparent variations between service settings be studied further
- that a similar study be conducted with other groups of mental health service users and in different geographical areas to determine what similarities and differences exist.

A draft of the final project report was forwarded to ForUs for their approval before it was sent for printing. This process did lead to some changes being made.

Dissemination

In keeping with a commitment to promote user involvement at all stages of the research, dissemination of this project took a variety of different forms. As noted above, a final project report was written and this was circulated to key service providers and other stakeholders. However, such a report is lengthy and thus perhaps not easily accessible to those who took part in the research. Therefore, a summary report was written, and this was widely circulated among the research sites and also within other user fora. The reports were also formally launched at an event hosted by the university (but organized jointly with ForUs) at which an invited audience of service users and service providers were presented with the key findings and the recommendations.

Other forms of dissemination that took place included the publication of papers (Northway et al. 2001b, 2001c; Davies et al. 2002; Parker and Northway 2002), two of which (Northway et al. 2001c; Parker and Northway 2002) were written collaboratively between university staff and representatives of ForUs. In addition, one joint conference presentation was given.

A key aim of the research was to inform the development of local policy and practice. To this end, members of ForUs discussed, as a group, the research report, the findings and the recommendations. They made the decision to formulate their own recommendations based on their analysis of the report and these were presented to the local joint health and social services planning group.

Outcomes

The starting point for this research was the desire of a group of mental health service users to undertake research in order to bring about a change in service provision. To this end they commissioned a piece of research but maintained ownership of both the process and the outcomes. The decision of ForUs to present their own analysis to the local planning group was an important element of their ownership of the research. What was most important was that their presentation of the research has led to some changes in practice.

However, outcomes were also evident in another context. As has been discussed, student nurses were involved in the study as data collectors. Since this was an innovative approach, it was felt essential to evaluate the preparation and support that was provided for them when undertaking this role. It was also recognized, though, that they had spent time in mental health service settings listening to the views and experiences of those who used the service. It was thus felt that any evaluation should ask about how the experience had influenced their views of user participation. As can be seen from the reflection below the study did impact on both their awareness and understanding of the research process as well as upon their perception of user involvement. As students commented:

> The participation in the research greatly emphasised the importance of service users' involvement into research and education and service development.

highlighted how little service user involvement there is.

(Davies et al. 2002)

Reflections of a student nurse

Involvement in the project had a number of positive outcomes for us as nursing students. First, it resulted in us having a greater awareness of the value of seeking service user's views on the services offered to them. Second, it gave us some insight into the challenges and complications that one might face both in designing the research tool and in gaining access to participants. Third, it enabled us to better link the theory of research to the practice of nursing. Additionally, it resulted in many of us improving our communication skills, which was beneficial to our practice generally. It also resulted in us being more aware of the importance of being able to provide services users with accurate information as to the medication they had been prescribed.

Although the project provided us with experience in only one approach to research, it resulted in us having both an increased interest in the research process and greater confidence in our ability to utilize and participate in research.

Linking theory and practice in collaborative research

Thus far, most of the discussion in this chapter has been descriptive or reflective with no reference to the wider literature concerning user involvement in research. It is thus important to address this deficit and to consider links between theory and practice in the context of this study.

At the time of undertaking this study, it was recognized that while the views of service users had been sought in other areas of health care historically this had tended not to be the case in the context of mental health services (Rogers et al. 1993). Even where their views had been sought, they had been placed in a very passive role leading to a feeling that research was being conducted on them rather than with them (Ramon 2000). Some participatory studies had been undertaken with mental health service users (e.g. Macleod 1997) but the number of such studies remained limited. Moreover, there was evidence that where mental health service users had raised concerns regarding their medication, or had asked for other forms of treatment, such requests had often been ignored (Holmes and Newnes 1996). It can, therefore, be seen that this study presented challenges both in respect of its methodology and its subject matter.

Some might argue that this study did not meet the requirements of participatory research since the actual study was undertaken by researchers based in an academic department rather than by a service user group themselves. However, in questioning the role of academics in participative research, Stoeker (1999) identifies three key roles. The first of these is as the initiator of research, the second as a consultant and the third as a collaborator. This research study would appear to come within the category of 'consultant' since here 'The community commissions the research, and the academic carries it out while being held accountable to the community' (Stoeker 1999: 844). He goes on to argue that such accountability can be 'intense' with the researcher seeking the input of the community at each stage of the study as was the case in this particular project.

Stoeker (1999) argues that communities may not wish to participate in every stage of the research process but does provide a framework by which it is possible to assess the extent of participation. He argues that there are six key decisional points that either the researcher or the community can control. The first is *defining the research question* and, in this study, ForUs had identified the key questions before commissioning the research. The task of the research team was, therefore, to refine the questions in collaboration with them. The second decisional stage is *designing the research*. Here, there was full involvement and the data collection tool was developed via piloting and discussion with ForUs. The third stage involves *implementing the research design* and here there was only minimal input from ForUs although regular feedback was given regarding progress. *Analysing the research data* was again primarily undertaken by the research team although subsequent analysis of the research report was also undertaken by ForUs in preparation for their presentation to service managers. The fifth decisional point is *reporting the research process* and here, as already been discussed, there was full engagement on the part of ForUs representatives. Finally, the sixth decision relates to *acting on the research results* and at this stage it can be seen that responsibility was taken by ForUs since they took action by seeking change from service providers.

There are some things that perhaps could have been done differently. For example, it would have been helpful to include more members of ForUs in the student preparation day. It was also recognized that there were limitations to the study in that it was conducted within one area and with people attending specific types of services. The findings, therefore, cannot be generalised to other users of mental health services or to other areas. However, using the framework proposed by Stoeker (1999) it can be seen that the study can be considered to be participative since power and control concerning key decisions rested with ForUs. It is also interesting to note that a more recent participatory research study, undertaken by a university based researcher and a group of mental health service users (Schneider et al. 2004), explored similar issues concerning medication, information and support. In contrast, in the later study reported by Schneider et al. (2004), service users were more actively involved in the research process rather than with decision making alone. This demonstrates the potential for future developments within this area.

The study also served to increase awareness of the potential for user involvement in research among student nurses. This is an important secondary gain in that it will, we hope, lay the foundations for greater use of participatory research within the health service.

Reflections of the project co-ordinator

This was a complex project to co-ordinate since it was important for ForUs to maintain ownership of the process. At times, this meant that decision making took some time but previous experience of participatory research had prepared me for this. However, an additional factor in this project was the involvement of student nurses as data collectors. As previously noted, this placed additional responsibilities upon myself and the research team since this was a development that I had not seen within other research studies. Nonetheless, it did provide a useful learning opportunity both for me and for the students. The research team needed to develop strategies that would ensure that students were adequately supported, and they had the opportunity to learn not only about research but also about user involvement. The outcomes achieved were worth the investment of both time and resources and some of the strategies used (such as the handbook and the 'on call' lecturer) might be used in future studies. I hope that this will increase the potential for more participatory research studies both by unlocking potential data collectors and by increasing awareness of this approach to research. In some senses, this may still be relatively uncharted territory but I would concur with the advice of Stoeker (1999) and encourage others to think about the possibilities, give it a shot, and learn from it.

Conclusion

This chapter has sought to provide an overview of one participatory research study that aimed not only to explore the views of mental health service users concerning the service they received but also to promote user involvement at all stages of the research process. This aim was generally achieved and while participation in some stages of the research process was more limited, this should not detract from the overall achievements.

In conclusion, it is perhaps fitting to end with a quote from one of the articles published as a result of the research since it sums up what we tried to achieve in the context of this research study:

> If user involvement is ever going to be more than gestures, and if balances of power are ever going to be addressed, service users must engage with the institutions of service providers, with the same tools and arguments they employ. Research is one way of doing this. However, the support of those with some experience in undertaking research partnerships is a route that ForUs found to be worth exploring.
>
> (Parker and Northway 2002: 116)

Acknowledgements

The authors would like to thank ForUs for the opportunity to work with them on this research project.

References

Davies, P., Lado, A., Northway, R., Bennett, G., Williams, R., Moseley, L. and Mead, D. (2002) 'An evaluation of student nurses' experiences of being a researcher in a mental health research project', *Nurse Education Today*, 22: 518–26.

Holmes, G. and Newnes, C. (1996) 'Medication – the holy water of psychiatry', *OpenMind*, November–December: 14–15.

Macleod, C. (1997) 'Research as intervention within community mental health', *Curationis: South African Journal of Nursing*, 20 (2): 53–6.

Northway, R. (1998) 'Oppression in the lives of people with learning difficulties: a participatory study', unpublished PhD thesis, University of Bristol.

Northway, R., Parker, M., Davies, P., Lado, A., Williams, R. and Moseley, L. (2001a) *Users of Mental Health Out-Patient Facilities, Day Hospitals and Day Centres in One County*

Borough: A Survey of their Experience of Medication and Other Therapies, Pontypridd, Wales: School of Care Sciences, University of Glamorgan.

Northway, R., Davies, P., Lado, A. and Williams, R. (2001b) 'Involving pre-registration students in a research project', *Nurse Researcher*, 8 (4): 53–64.

Northway, R., Parker, M. and Roberts, E. (2001c) 'Collaboration in research', *Nurse Researcher*, 9 (2): 75–83.

Parker, M. and Northway, R. (2002) 'The lion's cage', *OpenMind*, July–August: 116.

Ramon, S. (2000) 'Participative mental health research: users and professional researchers working together', *Mental Health Care*, 3 (7): 224–7.

Reason, P. (1998) 'Three approaches to participative inquiry', in N.K. Denzin and Y.S. Lincoln (eds) *Strategies of Qualitative Inquiry*, London: Sage.

Rogers, A., Pilgrim, D. and Lacey, D. (1993) *Experiencing Psychiatry: Users' Views of Services*, London: Macmillan in association with MIND.

Schneider, B., Scissons, H., Arney, L., Benson, G., Derry, J., Lucas, K., Misurelli, M., Nickerson, D. and Sunderland, M. (2004) 'Communication between people with schizophrenia and their medical professionals: a participatory research project', *Qualitative Health Research*, 14 (4): 562–77.

Stoeker, R. (1999) 'Are academics irrelevant? Roles for scholars in participatory research', *American Behavioural Scientist*, 42 (5): 840–54.

Index